DRAWING THE LINE

DRAWING THE LINE

Life, Death, and Ethical Choices in an American Hospital

SAMUEL GOROVITZ

New York   Oxford
OXFORD UNIVERSITY PRESS
1991

Oxford University Press

Oxford   New York   Toronto
Delhi   Bombay   Calcutta   Madras   Karachi
Petaling Jaya   Singapore   Hong Kong   Tokyo
Nairobi   Dar es Salaam   Cape Town
Melbourne   Auckland

and associated companies in
Berlin   Ibadan

Library of Congress Cataloging-in-Publication Data
Gorovitz, Samuel.
Drawing the line :
life, death, and ethical choices in an American hospital
/ Samuel Gorovitz.
p.   cm.   Includes bibliographical references (p.   ).
ISBN 0-19-504428-2
1. Medical ethics. 2. Hospital care—Moral and ethical aspects.
3. Beth Israel Hospital (Boston, Mass.)   I. Title.
R725.5.G67   1991   174′.2—dc20   90-7089

Portions of this manuscript have appeared previously in "Having a Heart for Barney Clark," *Los Angeles Times, January 14, 1983;* "Artificial Hearts: Questions to Ask and Not to Ask," *The Hastings Center Report,* October 1984; "Will We Still Be 'Human' If We Have Engineered Genes and Animal Organs," *The Washington Post,* December 9, 1984; "Preparing for the Perils of Practice," *The Hastings Center Report,* December 1984; "Bringing Senior Citizens on Line," *Technology Review,* January 1985; "Regulating the Advertising of Professional Success Rates," *Business and Professional Ethics Journal,* February 1985; "Ethical Issues in Long Term Care," in *The Impact of Technology on Long Term Care* (ed. J. Grana and D. McCallum, Project HOPE and the Office of Technology Assessment, 1986); "At the End of Life," *Syracuse Scholar,* Spring 1987; "Ethical Use of Fetal Tissue Transplants," *Syracuse Post-Standard,* February 23, 1989; and "Moral Conflict in Public Policy," *National Forum,* Fall 1989.

2 4 6 8 9 7 5 3 1

Printed in the United States of America
on acid-free paper

For Herman D. Stein

PREFACE

In May 1985, I began a seven-week visit at Boston's Beth Israel Hospital, then a 460-bed teaching hospital affiliated with the Harvard Medical School (and now at 504 beds). My official title was Visiting Scholar in Residence; unofficially, but perhaps more accurately, I was Authorized Snoop and Irritant-at-Large. During those seven weeks, my responsibilities were few and my opportunities great. I had come at the invitation of Beth Israel's president, Mitchell Rabkin, who provided me with ready access throughout the hospital. He asked only that I conduct a series of five weekly seminars for the hospital staff; this I happily did on the topic "Emerging Ethical Issues in Health Care."

I used the time primarily to learn as much as I could about life on the front lines of contemporary hospital care. That quest took me to meetings of many kinds—surgeons discussing the complications and mishaps of each preceding week; internists trying to map the best approach for dealing with a puzzling patient; nurses exploring ways to improve the continuity of patient care; administrative staff concerned about challenges to the hospital's financial integrity in an era of increasing competition in health care and of changing patterns of federal support; and many more. It also took me to the operating room, to intensive care units, to patients' rooms, to conversations about and with patients and their families. Wherever I went, I found an open responsiveness and a willingness to share uncertainties, fears, and frustrations as well as triumphs and gratifications.

These pages do not offer many conclusions about hospitals in general; it would make no sense to extrapolate from judgments about one rather unusual hospital to generalizations about others. I do not even presume to offer a comprehensive view of that one hospital. Medical sociology is not my field, and seven weeks is far too brief for any outsider to learn about more than a small proportion of what goes on in such a highly complex environment. But it is long enough to provide some valuable insights and a wealth of provocative experiences. The discussion revolves around three general themes. First, this is to some extent a partial portrait of day-to-day life as it is experienced in a particular hospital. Second, it is an examination of some ethical issues of concern within that hospital community. Third, this is an exploration of how those specific issues are related to larger questions of social policy. The discussion is heavily slanted, however, in the direction of issues I had already been thinking about and working on when I arrived at the hospital, supplemented by a selection of those that intrigued me most during my visit. This is therefore a very personal exploration of issues, highly idiosyncratic, and not intended to be comprehensive or systematic.

What goes on in hospitals, and the changing characteristics of the larger context of health care within which it goes on, are the focus of daily attention in American public life. The electronic and print media regularly feature medical issues, including technical, economic, ethical, and political aspects. Thoughtful essays about health care appear often in almost every serious, nonspecialized periodical, and new books about health care in America also surface almost weekly.

With such extensive scrutiny being brought to bear on medical matters, what justifies adding to the cascade of writings on such topics? Most of the issues discussed here are persistent, and have not changed in essential ways over the past few years. It is my hope that this book will provide a useful view of these issues that is not readily available elsewhere.

In some ways, this is a sequel to my earlier *Doctors' Dilemmas: Moral Conflict in Medical Care,** which, while a bit more scholarly in the traditional sense, is also addressed to a general audience. There, I emphasized various troubling aspects of the patient's

*Paperback edition, Oxford University Press, 1985.

experience with contemporary health care. Here, I have tried to reflect a much richer understanding of the professional lives of those who provide that care. My basic perspective remains the same; I still believe that good health care requires good communication between provider and patient in a climate of mutual respect, that we face major challenges and inevitable conflicts in seeking to provide such care in a just and affordable way, that conflict is best resolved by reasoned dialogue, that the modes of thought and reasoning traditional to the discipline of philosophy have much to contribute to such dialogue, and that it is an utter disgrace that we do not provide decent health care to the disadvantaged.

Over the past two decades, philosophers have played an increasingly prominent role in addressing the issues raised by modern medicine. That role, often controversial, has ranged from scholarship of a very traditional sort, focused on a general question (such as how scarce resources should be allocated or when patients should have the right to refuse life-sustaining treatment), to participation in the deliberations about what to do in a particular, ethically troubling, pending clinical case.

Although I am a philosopher, and although what I have said here is surely influenced by that fact, I do not see this book as a work within philosophy in any traditional sense. The boundaries of traditional disciplines are increasingly difficult to discern as interdisciplinary work gains in prominence and as the agendas and methodologies of traditional scholarship are themselves under increased critical scrutiny. Moreover, this is, by design, not a scholarly work, replete with references to the literature—nor does it provide a sustained argument in support of a single, focused thesis. (A brief guide to the scholarly literature appears as an appendix.) Instead, I have addressed it to the general reader who may be interested in a philosophically informed reflection on a diverse and interconnected array of intellectually compelling issues of great public concern, and who may also be intrigued, as I have been, by a deeper sense of the human experience of what goes on in hospitals.

I have written in two distinct voices, distinguished in the text by different typefaces. In one, I report on the events I witnessed and experienced at Boston's Beth Israel Hospital, as accurately as I can. That reporting is constrained by the reality of what happened in that time and in that place. But I also stand back from those events to consider the issues they raise and to discuss them in a way that is not limited by place or time, but instead follows the issues wherever they lead.

Those issues are diverse, but they raise a common set of questions: How should decisions be made, and by whom? What should be determined as a matter of law and what left a matter of judgment and discretion? Who should have access to what and at whose expense? How do those in health care learn what they need to know? What is the impact of computer-based information processing on health care? (I will return repeatedly to this topic.) What can we do to be more successful as patients, relatives of patients, or health care providers?

One kind of question interests me especially—the recurrent question of where to "draw the line." If there is any thematic unity to this work, it is an intermittent focus on how the distinction is made between the justified and the unjustified on the same continuum. How aggressively should a dying patient be treated? To what degree should patient autonomy be respected? How significantly should economic factors be allowed to influence health care decisions? When should a physician stop seeking more information, and make a judgment on the basis of the information that is available? There is no more pervasive or difficult question in health care than the question "How far should we go?" In various forms, it arises in every clinical unit of the hospital, in the business office, in the board room, and in the forums of health policy determination.

These matters concern us all in our various capacities as actual or potential patients, family members of the ill, purchasers of medical insurance, taxpayers, or health care providers. More fundamentally, they concern us as members of the human community, unavoidably involved in the evolution of a collective response to human illness and to modern modes of treating it.

Such complex questions resist definitive answers, and I have made no attempt here to put controversial questions to rest. I hope, however, to have shed some useful light on some of them and especially on how we can think constructively about them. Insofar as there is a thesis implicit in what I have said here, it is that the uncertainty that pervades health care today is of central significance to the making of sound decisions both at the personal and the policy levels, and that prior reflection on the issues at hand can facilitate the judgment that is called for in making such decisions well. To that end, I have addressed several issues and situations that can be expected to challenge us all for some time to come. Along the way, I hope also to have provided some practical advice about how physicians, patients and their families, and others concerned with health care can cooperate more effectively in service of the values they hold in common, both at the level of policy and at the level of individual clinical interactions.

My conviction that we must address these matters together—and that we have the capacity to do so constructively—antedates my visit to Boston's Beth Israel, but the way I think about them now has been greatly enriched by the events and perceptions of those seven weeks. I offer these reflections in order to share that enrichment more broadly.

Syracuse, N.Y.   S. G.
April 1990

ACKNOWLEDGMENTS

So many are due my thanks that it is impossible even to cite them, let alone do them justice. In Boston's Beth Israel Hospital, I was aided by many dozens, if not hundreds, of doctors, nurses, patients, family members, trustees, students, and staff members who granted me access to important and sometimes intimate dimensions of their lives. Mitchell T. Rabkin, the hospital's president, is owed the primary debt of gratitude; he conceived of my period of residence at the hospital, made and sustained the arrangements, and set the tone of the visit in an ideally constructive way. Among the many others who were exceptionally welcoming and helpful, the hospital chaplain, Rabbi Terry Bard, also merits special thanks.

Leona Schechter, my agent, provided much sound guidance, as did Susan Rabiner, who acquired the book at Oxford University Press. My students, in two classes, read portions of the emerging manuscript; useful suggestions were made by Erin Hill, David Harper, Sondra Ness, Rob Pietropaoli, and Julie Zito. The opportunity to present portions of the text at several universities led to further help from many voices in the ensuing discussions.

Two anonymous readers provided the publisher with excellent reports on the penultimate draft; I have followed their suggestions insofar as possible, and thank them, whoever they are. I am especially grateful to my editor at Oxford University Press, Valerie Aubry, for patience, encouragement, good advice, and the willingness to support a highly idiosyncratic project.

I appreciate the tolerance of Syracuse University's Vice Chancellor Gershon Vincow—who bore with unfailing good grace the news that I was at home writing on many occasions when I suspect he would have been pleased to find me in my office. My administrative secretary, Marcia Wisehoon, prepared the manuscript, including the index, with an enthusiasm that was itself a source of encouragement to complete the project.

The dedication bears the name of Herman D. Stein. Although he has no direct connection with this book, the tenacity to finish it was sustained by my awareness of the standard of accomplishment he has set. Social worker; scholar; educator; academic administrator; Borscht Belt comedian; management consultant to the computer industry; tireless worker, through the United Nations, in behalf of those in need throughout the Third World; mentor; friend; and inspiration—he has my thanks for enriching my sense of the valuable and expanding my sense of the possible.

Finally, as always, I am grateful for Judie, Heidi, and Eric Gorovitz—who always believed this project would be successfully completed, even when I did not.

CONTENTS

DRAWING THE LINE

.1.
. . .

INTRODUCTION

Any hospital is a complex community; Boston's Beth Israel especially so. Officially nonsectarian, in its history, leadership, and many aspects of its culture, it is a Jewish hospital. As a teaching affiliate of the Harvard Medical School, it is a Jewish hospital in a decidedly Protestant academic environment. It is located, however, in a largely Catholic political environment. And it is Jewish in a somewhat odd way. Its Board of Trustees, largely prominent members of the greater Boston business and professional community, was entirely Jewish until November 1989, as are most of its many substantial donors. But most of its patients and support staff are not. It is the hospital of choice for the Jewish community, but that community provides only a minority of the hospital's patient constituency. It is the hospital of choice for many others as well because it enjoys a reputation for leadership in providing sensitive, humane patient care. Yet as one of approximately thirty hospitals in the Boston area, it faces increasing competition for patients.

The hospital has its roots in the Mount Sinai Hospital Association, which sought in 1901 to establish a Jewish-sponsored facility "to give all Jews and non-Jews . . . all races, creeds and colors . . . Americans and non-Americans the benefit of our institution." That effort ultimately failed, but its supplies and equipment became part of the original inventory of the newly dedicated Beth Israel Hospital when it opened in 1916 in Roxbury. The Beth Israel Hospital also embraced the original values and objectives of the Mount Sinai Association. In August 1928, the hospital moved

3

to a new 200-bed facility on Brookline Avenue and began its affiliation with the nearby Harvard Medical School. In the intervening sixty years, it has grown to its present size of 504 beds. In addition to its in-patient capacity, it maintains an emergency unit and also operates an array of units for out-patient (ambulatory) care.

Any modern hospital exhibits many characteristics of a small city. It must have all the resources necessary to provide for the full range of needs of its patients and its staff, including communications systems, food services, building maintenance, waste disposal, and the like—it must even have independent power sources so that it can supply heat, light, and electricity to operate essential equipment in the event of a general failure of public utilities.

Because Boston's Beth Israel Hospital is a major teaching hospital, its complexity is greater still. Woven into the fabric of all it does are the Harvard medical students on clinical rotations, the house officers (young physicians in training in a residency program), and the clinical faculty who are the mentors of the students and house officers.

The staff physicians are organized into approximately two dozen clinical departments, ranging from Anesthesia, Behavioral Medicine, and Cardiology to Rheumatology, Radiology, and Surgery. The hospital's nursing staff of approximately 800, renowned for its central role in the provision of quality care, is based in twenty-nine nursing stations supported by a central nursing administration. Ambulatory care encompasses nearly fifty different units, with such specialties as audiology, hypertension, pain-management, sexual dysfunction, sleep disorders, and infectious diseases contracted by travellers.

The various clinical activities are supported by dozens of additional departments of professional staff, ranging from the angiography suite and the animal research facility, through the library and laboratories (of which there are forty), to the office of utilization review and the video production center. An infrastructure for all the professional activity is maintained by a large and diverse organization of support staff in admitting and in accounts receivable, in the laundry and in nutrition services, in paging, parking, payroll, printing and purchasing, in records, security, and a great deal more.

The diversity of the hospital's activities is mirrored in its physical premises. Hospitals tend to be architecturally complex; Boston's Beth Israel is especially so, comprising sixteen buildings, each with its own name, linked in various ways at various angles and levels. Because the hospital has grown over the decades, its buildings range from new to over sixty years old. Construction workers are always on the scene, and change is constant. If the hospital is not putting up a new building at any given moment, it is renovating older spaces.

Within its walls, the hospital provided 159,433 patient days in 1985—a patient day being one patient staying in the hospital for one day. (If the 460 beds had all been filled for all 365 days of the year, the number of patient days would have been 167,900. So the occupancy rate was well over 90%—very high indeed.) Almost a dozen newborns a day were delivered in the hospital. Counting these newcomers, there were 24,395 admissions (so the average length of stay was just under a week). Surgery was performed 9,846 times—nearly three dozen cases each weekday.

The ambulatory units also maintained a brisk pace, with over 173,000 visitors—nearly 500 a day. This includes the almost 35,000 callers at the emergency room—one for every fifteen minutes, day and night, all year long.

The treatment of these patients was supported by more than 87,000 X rays and well over a million laboratory tests. And the cost of the hospital's activities, including $16.5 million in research expenditures, was just short of $150 million. Of that total, less than one million came from direct charitable contributions; about $5 million more came from endowment and investment income. Most of the rest—more than $130 million—came directly from patient revenues.

Administering such an institution is rather like conducting a leading orchestra with no time between concerts for rehearsals. Changes occur in the staff from time to time, and members of the audience come and go, but the music must continue without missing a beat day or night, and the repertoire must always include the full range of works by the *avant garde* composers as well as the best of the classics.

Having grown up in the Boston area and lived there until going to graduate school, I had many occasions to visit friends and relatives in Beth Israel. Those visits were always brief and focused not on the hospital as an institution but on the well-being of a particular patient. I thus returned to the hospital in 1985 as one to whom it was familiar, yet largely unknown.

Seven weeks in residence did not give me a thorough understanding of anything in the hospital, nor even a minimal glimpse of all its many parts and functions. But I had enough of a look to get a rough sense of the enterprise as a whole, and to gain a keen awareness of the fascinating problems that are a part of the daily life there. It is those problems, as they involve difficult decisions and ethical challenges, that I am primarily concerned about here, because they are shared by health care settings throughout the country. My focus is thus on Boston's Beth Israel Hospital as the particular context in which I considered these problems, but the problems themselves constitute the larger agenda.

Hospitals have become more systematically interested in such issues in recent years, individually and collectively. For example, in 1983 the American Hospital Association established a Special Committee on Biomedical Ethics, which issued its report, *Values in Conflict: Ethical Issues in Hospital Care*, a few months before my arrival at Boston's Beth Israel. The authors of that report raised many questions of broad social policy, concerning such matters as how access to health care should be assured and at whose expense, how health care needs should be compared with other social needs, and how basic medical research should be funded.

They also raised more directly clinical issues, such as the distinction between the prolongation of life and the prolongation of dying, the need to find ways to ensure that advances in medical science will be applied wisely, the need to enhance the patient's role in clinical decision making, and the economic conflict between establishing a costly organ transplantation program and allocating increased resources to the more common unmet health needs of the hospital's community.

When such matters arise as particular conflicts in a specific health care setting, the necessary decisions are sometimes made within the community of patients, family, and health care workers. But, increasingly, there is also a strong presence either of lawyers and judges, or at least of an awareness that the legal and judicial systems are potential participants if the matter is not congenially resolved. The report expresses concern about how the fear of legal liability can influence clinical and administrative decisions, and raises questions about the relationship between those decisions and the proper role of the courts.

Recognizing that the various issues they address are matters of broad public concern, the report's authors declare that "Hospitals cannot be passive in the face of such dilemmas," but must instead "Take the lead in drawing national attention to issues that should be discussed and debated openly in the broadest public policy arenas." How would such issues be revealed in the day-to-day life of patients and staff in the hospital? Would they be going about their business with a narrow focus on the clinical problem of the moment, essentially undistracted by the larger questions? Or would these larger issues keep intruding? How would health care providers deal with the constant necessity of making difficult choices in a hospital setting, as they confronted individual cases one by one?

Apart from the few seminars I was scheduled to present, it was my intention to enter the hospital not primarily as an educator, seeking to raise issues, or as a consultant, helping to resolve them, but as an observer, trying to discover what issues naturally arise and learn how they are addressed in this one hospital. Since many issues that concerned the American Hospital Association's committee did arise in what I heard and saw, sometimes explicitly and sometimes implicitly, it is my hope that this collection of perceptions and reflections will make a constructive contribution to that broad public discussion.

.2.

THE
INITIAL
VISIT

B ecause of my earlier work on ethical issues in medicine, I was invited to present a guest lecture at Boston's Beth Israel Hospital several years ago. Some of that work had explored ways in which patients can be the victims of insensitivity on the part of their doctors. I had concluded that much about being a patient is not generally well understood by physicians. This sense of distance between doctors and physicians, despite the intimacy of their interactions, was supported by my dabbling in amateur anecdotal sociology.

When I spoke to a large, nonmedical, adult audience, I would often ask a series of simple questions. First, "How many of you have been treated for a serious illness? I don't mean that you have seen a doctor for a routine matter, but that you have had surgery or have been hospitalized for some other significant reason, or have in some other way seriously been a patient." The older the audience, the larger the percentage who responded positively. I then addressed those who had such experience.

"However much you may trust, admire, and appreciate your doctor, how many of you have as a patient experienced some aspect of your medical care—of what your doctor did—that was not merely disappointing or discomforting, but was deeply offensive to you, that struck you as an enraging violation of your dignity or in some way made you feel betrayed or abused?" The smallest positive response I have ever seen to that question was about 80% of those with experience as patients. Often it was substantially higher. Again, I addressed the next question to those who had just responded positively.

"Did you discuss your distress with anyone at all—spouse, friend, neighbor?" Typically, the same set of hands goes up; people who have had such unpleasant experiences rarely keep silent about them. Then, one last question.

"How many of you, at the time or later, discussed, mentioned, or in any other way communicated your discontent to the physician about whom you had the complaint?" The largest positive response I have seen to this last question was about 17% of the previous respondents; often it is much smaller! I concluded that patients commonly have complaints about at least some aspects of what their physicians do, but they typically do not reveal those complaints to their physicians. It is no surprise, given the immense differential in power and authority between a doctor and a sick patient who looks to the doctor with a mix of fear, hope, awe, and dependency. Doctors, I thought, would be very interested in this.

In each course I teach, I grade my students; they must also grade me. I ask them, in the process, to indicate anonymously what they would most like to see changed about the course or the instructor. There is rarely anything new to me in those evaluations after all these years, but I do still learn something useful from them once in a while. Such evaluation of faculty by students is common in academic life.

A doctor could do the same sort of thing, trying to find out in some nonthreatening way what his or her patients liked least about their experience. That should be useful to any doctor wanting to provide more satisfying medical care. I once mentioned this idea to a prominent oncologist. He replied that he didn't need evaluations from his patients. "My patients love me," he affirmed.

"I'm sure they do," I replied, "and probably for good reason. But couldn't you still learn something by asking what they *don't* like about your practice?"

"No," he responded, "they're not discontent." I asked how he could be so certain. "Well," he answered, "they're not complaining."

Intrigued, I wrote an editorial about mutual misunderstanding in medical care. One paragraph said:

> Even the best doctors, given all the pressures that they must bear, could benefit from more structured ways of remaining informed about how their efforts are viewed by their patients. That, combined with a greater public understanding of how hard it is to practice the physician's fallible art, could benefit both parties. Such mutual understanding might lead to more effective surveillance of the quality of medical practice and a lessened tendency on the part of the patients to rush to the courts in anger and frustration.

The *Los Angeles Times* ran the piece under the headline "Medical Profession Faces an Important Selling Job: Customer Relations."

The medical director of a hospital in Southern California wrote to me, endorsing the idea, and asking for examples of successful efforts by physicians to get such patient evaluations. I had none to provide, so I telephoned several others who might know about such things. In the end I had to admit complete failure to find anyone who knew of a physician who had ever tried such a measure. And when I later tried to persuade a group of academic physicians at a leading medical school that it might be worth trying, just as an experiment to discover whether doctors might gain useful information by such systematic inquiry, I was stunned by the resistance—by the fact that people who claimed to be dedicated to empirical inquiry and the ways of science could explicitly dismiss my idea as *obviously* not worth trying, on the ground that it was known in advance that nothing useful to doctors could result. (I have since learned of a few instances of physicians who do conduct such inquiries.)

This experience reinforced my sense that doctors and patients are isolated from one another more than they realize. It also heightened my curiosity about what it is like to be a physician—about what sorts of problems and pressures sustain their distance and separateness, and make it so hard for them to be open to new ideas from outside their profession. How do they deal with the uncertainties, expectations, and decisions that confront them, and at what personal cost? How do they learn, and keep learning, what they need to know? I began to turn my attention away from the problems patients have with their doctors, and toward the problems that doctors have—toward how the experience of providing medical care affects the lives and welfare of the providers.

With surprise and alarm, I learned that medicine is a hazardous profession—that hundreds of doctors each year are lost to the profession because of alcoholism, drug addiction, and suicide. These phenomena, collectively known as physician impairment, are part of the dark side of medical practice—little discussed in the training of physicians or among the public, but widespread problems within the profession.

About twenty years ago, I knew a doctor who seemed to be one of life's winners. He was a successful and respected member of the medical community, had a lovely, loving wife and three fine children, and was viewed with affection and admiration by friends, patients, and colleagues alike. But he shot himself. At the time, I thought his suicide inexplicable. Only much later did I learn of the frequency of such tragic events.

I had long argued that the deficiencies of medical education were detrimental to the interests of patients, that medical schools were devoting insufficient attention to the cultivation of those sensitivities and cognitive capacities that are essential to the highest quality medical care. Recent studies from within the medical world supported this view, and a report by the Association of American Medical Colleges concluded in 1984 that medical education was in serious need of major reform. But if there was general agreement that the character of medical education was bad for patients, was it not also worth asking how well it served the interests of physicians?

I read the literature on physician impairment, noting that published estimates of the number of impaired American physicians range from a low of 12,000 to a high of over 50,000! By any measure, this is a serious public health problem even without beginning to consider the inferior medical care that results. (For comparison, there are about 30,000 victims of cystic fibrosis and 21,000 patients with hepatitis B.) Although this extensive literature showed increasing concern with the identification and treatment of impaired physicians, it had little to say about preventing impairment in the first place. (Perhaps this is merely a reflection of the medical profession's general tendency to find treatment a more compelling prospect than prevention.)

All these articles contained only a few scattered calls for efforts on the part of medical schools to anticipate the problems of impairment, and even fewer reports of such efforts. In a classic article on the subject, George Vaillant and his colleagues, in 1970, had argued that "Medical schools must assume greater responsibility for teaching their students that they represent a high-risk population for drug abuse, and that, unchecked, the virtues of the good physician can increase the risk." And Julien Mendlewicz and Jean Wilmotte, a year later, wrote, "Since physicians and medical students are well identified as a high risk suicide group, preventive efforts should be built into the medical school curricula. . . . Medical students should be encouraged to confront themselves through thoroughgoing introspection of their own approach to life." Yet, as late as 1983, Brian Doyle found that only six of twenty leading medical schools claimed any formal planning concerning student mental health needs, and he and David Cline called for reforms "to maximize the value of medical student education to prevent the impairment of physicians."

I also read the various reports calling for reformation of medical education. Although there is occasional mention of the stress of being a medical student or a physician in training, I was surprised by the silence of these reports on the matter of impairment among the ranks of practicing doctors. I concluded that physicians are not just somewhat isolated from some of the thoughts and feelings of their patients, they are also distanced from some of the realities of their own lives as physicians. This perception, too, increased my desire to gain a deeper understanding of those realities.

In April 1984, I had the privilege of delivering the 16th annual Dr. Nathan Sidel Lecture on the Art of Medicine at Boston's Beth Israel Hospital. Dr. Sidel, in whose honor the series had been established, was a distinguished clinician in Boston, admired for his wisdom and integrity. I looked forward to seeing him in the hospital, but he died a few months before the event. In preparing the lecture, I was keenly aware of his concern for the training of humane physicians. His family would be present, and we would all feel his absence acutely. I decided not to talk about patients at all, but to focus on the welfare of physicians. The title of the lecture was "Why Medical Education Is Bad For Doctors."

It should be no surprise that physicians often fall victim to the stresses of practice, or that medical education should be judged as inadequate to the demands of the time. Current health care is marked by the pervasive presence of high technology; increasing fragmentation of services; widespread concern about the high incidence of malpractice claims and their impact on insurance rates and on the character of clinical decisions; increasingly strained relations between providers and patients, nurses and doctors, participants in health care and third-party payers, and even between those responsible for clinical education and their colleagues who are responsible for the associated clinical facilities; the distorting impact of national for-profit corporations on the structure of health care; and more. Throughout, in these times of fetal tissue transfer, withdrawal of artificial nutrition and hydration, technically assisted reproduction, genetic therapy, organ transplantation, and all the rest, moral anxiety becomes more prevalent almost daily as medical progress raises new questions about what is right to do. Physicians often have the feeling of being under seige in the face of these diverse pressures within the profession and in the glare of heightened critical scrutiny from outside the profession.

Let's consider two illustrative cases. The first is that of Dr. A. He finds that he is spending more time than ever before dealing with decisions he was never trained to make—decisions at the edges of life, where the question is not what can be done for the patient, but whether medical skills are worth using. He is acutely uncomfortable when the issue turns from how to sustain a patient's life to such questions as whether to stop providing nutrition and hydration, thereby to end a patient's life. But such questions crowd in on him more and more.

He is aware of the failings and errors of some of his faltering colleagues and is increasingly troubled by his responsibility regarding their behavior. Some of them have been his colleagues for years, or perhaps even his friends. He sees them and thinks, "There but for the grace of God go I." Yet he remains silent about their errors at his own growing peril. His insurance rates are soaring, his patients are becoming more assertive, the government is becoming more meddlesome, the insurance paperwork gets steadily worse, and he feels as though he is losing control of that one main part of his life where he had it. Perhaps he even has to endure the scrutiny of philosophers whose unwelcome inquiries occasionally cut rather close to the bone.

His children have left the fold; they're off to college—rather suddenly, it seems. Sadly, he realizes that he never found the time to get to know them very well. Even his wife is straining at the bit. With the children gone from home, she's taken on a decidedly feminist tone, disturbing his comfortable confidence in the old patterns of support and authority. All in all, he finds less and less gratification in the treadmill he has been on for twenty-five years.

His despair deepens as he falls victim to the Imposter Syndrome—the loss of self-esteem that attends the belief that one is pretending to a role one cannot actually fill. His long-standing social drinking gets heavier. He turns to Demerol in quest of tranquility, and then, one day, is found in his office, dead of an overdose.

The second case is simpler to describe. Dr. B has been trained at a leading, research-oriented medical school, to an exceedingly high standard of clinical performance, which she has internalized. She believes that one should not have children unless one can meet comparably high standards of parental competence. She also believes that she cannot meet both sets of standards. After agonizing deliberation, she reluctantly concludes that she cannot in good conscience become a mother. But her intense desire to have children does not fade.

Dr. A is a composite of real cases. The story is fictional, yet medical people readily recognize in it someone they have known. Dr. B is real. Perhaps the excruciating role conflict she experienced is an example of the factors that yield a suicide rate for women in medicine that is on the order of three times that for men.

There followed a series of decidedly unflattering remarks about medical education—about how it proceeds apace essentially as in the past, paying no central regard to the fact that its alumni are at serious risk. And how has it proceeded?

It is commonplace by now that good medical practice requires acknowledging the full humanity of the patient. The proper focus of the doctor's attention is not a disease or organ system, it is a person—who perhaps has a disease or a troublesome organ system. If one hangs around the wards a bit one can still hear reference to "the kidney in 342" or the "bypass in 340," but that is loose talk. Everyone acknowledges that the responsibility of doctors is to treat the person, and thus to have a sense of who that person is—including an awareness of the values and aspirations of the patient, and not merely an awareness of the physiological facts. This point gains assent even from physicians who are narrow in their focus and callous in their approach to patients. It is by now so much a part of the culture of medicine that it cannot be denied.

The directly analogous point about medical students, however, seems hardly to have been noticed. Medical schools process their raw material—incoming pre-medical students—through what is called "professionalization," into medical practitioners and researchers, as if they were unaware that, like patients, medical students are persons too. I am not referring here to the often noted and lamented obsession in medical education with a narrow factual and clinical focus, but to something worse. Medical education often encourages imprudent role modeling, and there is even documented evidence that medical students, in their clinical years, are often subjected to abuse that goes well beyond the imposition of rigorous and demanding standards of performance. Worst of all, medical schools typically just try to turn the pre-medical students into doctors; in so doing they are insensitive to the problems of leading a successful life—as a spouse, parent, neighbor, and citizen—into which life the practice of good medicine is successfully and harmoniously integrated.

Even when the doctors' problems of adjustment have been addressed in medical schools, it has been in a way that takes the context of medical practice as given, and seeks a happier accommodation to that context. The focus is on stress management, rather than on possible modifications of those conventions of practice that exacerbate stress. This simply reinforces the students' perception that those conventions are fixed and immutable.

So even stress management training has an aspect that is repressive and unhealthful.

Instead, medical students should be induced by their educations to cultivate the habit of stepping back from the daily grind to reflect on and reassess their goals, their patterns of interaction with others, and the institutions in which they participate. They should learn the importance of periodically transcending the parochialism of their own most familiar patterns of experience. It should also be a fundamental part of medical education, training, and even practice to address the kinds of questions that go beyond medical fact, but which are a vital part of the fabric of every medical life:

Having promised to hear his son's tuba solo at the junior high school band concert, a physician is running late at the office. A non-emergency walk-in patient, not previously under the physician's care, is very upset at the prospect of being turned away. But his son had been very upset when his father failed to appear at the last concert, having said he would be there. How should the physician deal with such conflict?

Two people are discussing with a doctor the treatment of their aged, rapidly failing relative, for whom they have custody. Sharp, emotional, acrimonious disagreement emerges between them about how treatment should proceed. How should the doctor respond?

A physician suspects that her colleague is beset by personal problems. He seems to be drinking more heavily in social settings and is behaving somewhat erratically in nonclinical situations. There is no hard evidence of malpractice or deterioration in quality of care, but there are discomforting rumors that he has been careless with some recent patients. What is the physician's first responsibility? How should she think about whether and how to intervene?

I emphasized that myriad similar problems confront doctors at every stage of a medical career. They concern the management of time, the uses of leisure, the ability to adapt to changing circumstances in health care and in other dimensions of life, and more.

Feeling increasingly like a haranguing cleric, and with substantial misgivings about how my diatribe was striking an essentially medical audience, I continued.

The physician's ability to deal gracefully with these inevitable problems will depend largely on the extent to which he or she has a clear and coherent set of values and on how those values affect the decisions that must be made both within the practice of medicine and within the larger life of which that practice is a part—albeit a central part. For this reason, physicians should cultivate the habit of reflective reassessment of their profession and their relation to it. Medical education should teach them to ask repeatedly: how does the way I lead my life conform to what I know about leading healthy successful lives? But medical education does not prompt such reflection except in superficial and tokenistic ways. . . .

The interests of physicians will not be fully respected until medical education acknowledges the humanity of future physicians in all its dimensions and all its diversity. Medical education should prepare them to deal with the moral and personal conflicts they will inevitably face. It should teach them to accept with grace and candor both their own limitations and those of their profession. It should represent to them honestly not just the glories but the perils of medical practice.

Until this becomes a standard feature of medical education, medical schools will continue to send their alumni forward as innocents, seeing themselves embarked on a path of service and affluence, but unwittingly directed all too often toward drink, drugs, dysfunction, despair, and death. . . .

Physicians are not alone in having a high rate of impairment; other high stress occupations also have such problems, and their professional schools also omit any serious address to such issues. But even if impairment rates for doctors were no higher than those of lawyers, corporate executives, or others, at most that observation would show that the need for reformation of professional education is not restricted to medicine. At the heart of the matter is the fact that our professional schools have primarily been training institutes for the development of a particular set of advanced vocational skills. But the times have caught up with that sort of training and passed it by, and the victims are many. To set the matter right will take nothing less than making professional education the new agenda of our professional schools. Until that happens, medical education will continue to be bad for doctors.

There followed a lively and well-informed discussion, and the response was certainly gracious. But I had to leave immediately after the lecture. I had offered a bitter pill, it seemed to me, and regretted having to depart with no secure sense of how well my audience took it. Happily, I received a letter a short time later from Mitchell Rabkin, the hospital's president. He had concluded that the sort of outside perspective I had offered could be stimulating to staff in the hospital, and he knew that I stood to learn greatly from a close and sustained look at life in the medical trenches. He raised the question of my visiting the hospital for an extended period of time, and we worked out the details. I was delighted to have an opportunity to witness the playing out of issues I had been concerned with for several years. In May 1985 I arrived to take up residence for about two months as an outsider on the inside.

.3.
THE
FIRST
WEEK

My first few days at the hospital were mainly days of introduction. I met various members of the hospital staff—physicians, nurses, business people—and all assured me of their interest and cooperation. In the process, I began to learn my way around the labyrinth.

To get to my next appointment, I leave my office in the administrative area and go to another building via an underground tunnel. Along the way, I see a worker briskly moving a heavy load of medical supplies in the opposite direction. He greets me, in a marked Spanish accent, with a cheerful "Good morning." I make a few turns, following signs and looking for the elevator, and then give up. I find a maintenance worker mopping the floor. There is an odd enthusiasm about him; he is not just moving his mop around, he seems very much to want the floor to be clean. I ask directions; he takes a few steps to the next corridor and points to the elevator.

Some hospitals are dank and gloomy; some, like this one, are bright and pleasant. I realize that good medical care is possible in both types of surroundings, and that a hospital, like a university, must be judged primarily on the basis of the people within it and the quality of their interactions (assuming appropriate technical

19

capacities.) Still, drab and shabby surroundings inhibit achieving the best in education, and I am confident also that the aesthetic environment in a hospital is medically relevant. So I am pleased that Boston's Beth Israel is a pretty place—that the graphics on the walls prompt one to stop with admiration, that the waiting areas are attractive and inviting, that the staff seem happy with the environment they work in. At the same time, I realize, even on this first day, that my experience here will not tell me much about life in other hospitals—especially in some of the dismal old hospitals I have seen.

On the third day, I attend a dinner at the Harvard Club for some hospital trustees and an assortment of senior members of the medical and nursing staffs. We meet in the Aesculapian Room and mingle, amidst the dark wood and oil paintings, over drinks and hors d'oeuvres. Above the fireplace hangs a portrait of Aesculapius; on the far wall are the images of sixteen medical greats, including Oliver Wendell Holmes, from the nineteenth century; elsewhere, the burning of Charlestown in 1775, and two renditions of the Harvard Medical School—1883 and 1963. Looking around the room, I recall a recent visit to the original Asclepion.

The Asclepion (named for Asclepius, son of Apollo and Coronis, who became the Greek god of medicine) is the site, on the Island of Cos in the Eastern Aegean Sea, where Hippocrates is said to have taught at the first medical school. From the Hippocratic Center of Cos—recently developed by a medical foundation as a site for conferences and related activities, one can look out through peaceful olive groves, across a narrow stretch of sea, to the Turkish coast. And if one can forget for a moment the hostile relations between Greece and Turkey, it is possible in that tranquil and isolated spot almost to imagine that one is back in the ancient days of Hippocrates.

Nearby, at the ruins of the Asclepion, young Greek students re-enact the ceremony—at least as they imagine it—of a medical student solemnly taking the Oath of Hippocrates. To the sound of a wooden flute, in carefully measured steps, a procession of toga-clad youth slowly descends a long stone staircase to the level ground below, where maidens sprinkle flower petals on the new physician.

At the base of the stairs, he recites the ancient oath in Greek; after the ceremony the visitors are each given a scroll with an English translation. Some of what the oath provides remains uncontroversial to this day: "I will follow that system of regimen which, according to my ability and judgment, I consider for the benefit of my patients and abstain from whatever is deleterious and mischievous." It also prohibits the seduction of patients and the violation of confidentiality. But other provisions have long since been abandoned, such as the requirement to teach the art of medicine to the children of other physicians "without fee or stipulation" if they wish to learn it. And some provisions are at the heart of current controversy—the prohibitions against abortion and against providing advice on request about lethal medicines.

The oath has been part of the tradition of medical practice for millennia. But it dates from far simpler times, and it has come under heavy attack of late, both as being inadequate to the problems of the day, and even as embodying moral precepts that are substantively indefensible. These criticisms have become so severe that some medical schools no longer administer the oath as part of their commencement ceremony. For example, in 1985, the graduating class at the Pennsylvania State University College of Medicine, judging the oath as "not an adequate expression of feelings, goals, or moral commitment," designed a ceremony of its own, featuring a covenant between physician and patient, rather than any affirmation on the part of the new physicians alone (*Annals of Internal Medicine* 1985:103:941–43).

The choices and challenges faced by today's doctors, and the reality of their complex relationships with patients, peers, and social situations, have left the Hippocratic oath behind. A disarming innocence and simplicity mark the re-enactment at Cos; watching that peaceful ceremony in the warm Aegean breeze, one can only wonder what Hippocrates would think today of his professional descendants and their current plight.

The scene in the Aesculapian Room is somewhat kaleidoscopic; many people here are among the dozens I have met in the last three days, and I struggle to put names to the faces I recognize and assimilate the names I am hearing anew.

It is always good for trustees to meet with those who do an organization's work, so I note with satisfaction that, around me in the room, lawyers, bankers, business executives, and other trustees are talking not with their own numbers, but with doctors and nurses. At dinnertime, we are seated at four tables, carefully mixed, it seems, to ensure professional diversity.

We introduce ourselves around the tables, and resume our conservations; moments later Dr. Rabkin rises, taps on a glass, and gives us our instructions. There is no such thing as a free meal, he reminds us, and proceeds to set the task that will earn us our dinners. He introduces me formally to the group, explains the nature of my association with the hospital, and then instructs us to identify and discuss over dinner what we see as the most worrying ethical problems in medicine and health policy for the coming few years. One person at each table is appointed as recorder.

During the dinner, the conversation was lively and wide-ranging. I refrained from addressing our charge explicitly, believing it most important to learn from others what they think the problems are. And I did not want to be cast into the role of "ethics expert" as if I could somehow tell them what their moral anxieties should be. They had plenty to say; I limited my participation to probing and trying to clarify the views they expressed.

At the end of the meal, Dr. Rabkin rose again and called on the recorders at each table in turn to tell us what their groups had to say. There was almost no overlap among the four reports. Each table had a somewhat different mix of professions, and each conversation had gone its own way. One list emphasized the impact of economic constraints and marketing realities on health care decisions, another the distorting impact on clinical practice of concern about professional liability. Some expressed particular interest in the consequences of new techniques of human reproduction, new understanding of genetics, new ways of screening and sorting people with respect to health risks. Others had been thinking about decisions at the end of life—about the demographics of an aging society and our growing capacity to sustain the lives of those who are very ill and very old. They were all good lists, full of challenging questions, and welcome proof that my interest in such questions was broadly shared within the hospital community. And the hospital is very much a community.

Each week, the president's office publishes two newsletters for the staff. One is called "Dear Doctor." The first issue since my arrival welcomes me, announces the series of lectures I will give, and notes my office and telephone number. So my shingle is hung. The doctors have now been told that there is a philosopher in residence, but it remains to be seen whether there is any business.

The other newsletter is called "Newsletter for Employees," and goes to nonmedical staff. I pick up a copy for my file. It, too, tells of my visit. Later, passing the information desk in the lobby, I notice three stacks of the newsletter. I reach for another copy; to my surprise, it is in French. I look at the next stack; it is in Spanish. In the president's office, I ask why the newsletter is distributed in three languages. The administrative assistant says, "Dr. Rabkin has them translated every week. Some of the staff are more comfortable in those languages than in English." I remember that worker, in the underground passage, with the Spanish accent.

Later, I see Dr. Rabkin in the hall; we're going up the stairwell together. I mention my sense that the staff have an unusual degree of commitment to the purposes of the hospital; they seem to feel themselves part of a common enterprise whatever their station or task. Earlier, there have been labor problems here; at one time there was conflict and even litigation about possible union activity. Perhaps undercurrents of conflict remain. But on the surface, at least, there's a remarkable sense of collective endeavor.

I applaud the sensitivity reflected in the translation of the newsletter, but Dr. Rabkin shrugs off the remark. We pass a worker in the stairwell, wiping a wall. Dr. Rabkin tells me of how he once had some young doctors dress in the uniforms of maintenance staff and move about the hospital to get a feel for how the support staff are perceived and treated. "Anyone can wash a wall," he notes. "That's easy. The trick is to get it clean."

The hospital is organized in many different ways for different purposes. There are various departments divided by medical categories—surgery, medicine, radiology, orthopedics, etc. There are other clinical services as well, such as nursing, physical therapy, and social work. Sustaining their collective efforts is a large assortment of support services ranging from the program-mers who work on the hospital's extensive computerized systems for patient records and medical research to the transportation workers who move patients from place to place in wheelchairs or on carts.

At the same time, many others must tend to the business side of health care, which grows more complicated daily. So there are departments concerned with billing, fund-raising, public rela-tions, and the like. And the secure and effective functioning of the physical facilities, so easily taken for granted by providers and patients alike, depends on legions of staff who strive to keep the sixteen buildings all in good working order, amidst the unceasing activity of renovation here and new construction there. It all comes together in the patient care units, each of which depends on a vast assortment of departments and services in the hospital. Whether it is 7F or 4N matters little; each is a microcosm of the larger whole; in each, dozens of different functions support the care of each patient. The structure of patient care units therefore cuts across the other structures of hospital organization. A prob-lem or deficiency in any one of those can show up in a patient's room. And, although the hospital must have its financial affairs in order, the bottom line that counts most is found in the patients' rooms.

I naturally wanted to spend some time in the patient care units. Instead of my visiting many of them, however, it was arranged for me to affiliate primarily with one in order to get a sense of continuity over time. My unit was 4N, a general medical unit. Some of the patients in 4N came in via the emergency room; some had been released from intensive care; some were admitted for testing, diagnosis, and treatment. A few would go on to a surgical or other specialty unit. Most would recover and go home. Some would die.

Each morning at eleven the medical staff of 4N gathered for what are called "visit rounds." The group included a senior physician, residents, interns (in essence, first-year residents), and medical students doing a clerkship in the department of medicine. It was never clear to me or anyone I asked whether these sessions are called visit rounds because they are often presided over by a clinician visiting from outside the hospital—an attending physician with a clinical appointment in the medical school, referred to as "the Visit," or because part of the process includes going around to visit patients. Etymology is not a major concern in hospitals.

We meet at 11 A.M. in a small, crowded conference room in 4N, a general medical unit. The room is uncomfortable, with more furniture than one can gracefully walk around but less than will accommodate the group. Visit rounds begin with a report by a medical resident on the new admissions. It has been a quiet night and morning; nothing dramatic is afoot. The Visit turns to the house officers.

"Who's got a case?" he asks. Most of the house officers have index cards—in their hands, their pockets, on the table in front of them. There's a very brief bit of shuffling around, looking at cards and at one another. Then an intern volunteers a case. He describes a patient, reviewing the history briefly and reporting on current status. The talk is full of language I don't understand—reports of lab tests and physical observations. Another resident comes in and sits down as the presentation continues.

A beeper sounds. Two residents reach for their little black boxes—it is impossible to tell immediately whose beeper is sounding. Both of the boxes are tapped, then one of them emits a mix of static and a voice giving a telephone extension. The resident who has been called leaves the room to answer the page; a moment later another resident joins the group. A nurse opens the door, looks around, and leaves. A young man, without comment, comes in and retrieves a book from the room. The scene seems to have much the same sort of choreography as a Marx Brothers film, but the doctors maintain their concentration on the case despite the constant coming and going.

The intern continues, "The patient was felt to be more alert this morning. . . ." This use of a passive construction—conventional in the context of medical charts—strikes me as odd. By whom, I wonder.

The Visit leads a discussion of the case, skillfully asking the younger doctors for opinions, drawing them out, guiding them, giving his opinions in the end about the proper management of the case. I have no sense here of hierarchy; the students freely ask questions and the Visit corrects errors in a kindly fashion.

Several more cases are discussed; then the Visit says, "Well, let's have a look."

There are rounds, and there are grand rounds. Going around from room to room to see patients is called rounds. Surgeons sometimes go on rounds very early in the morning, before going to the operating rooms. A patient recovering from surgery may well be awakened at six by the surgical team; on a medical floor the internists might not be around until eleven. So there are rounds going on somewhere much of the time. It is a basic part of the doing of medicine in the hospital.

The entourage that does the looking typically includes an attending physician who has a clinical appointment to the faculty, a few house officers—residents and interns, some medical students who are doing a clinical rotation on that service, and one or more nurses working on the case. In a teaching hospital, the attending physician is central to the picture, framed and matted by the rest of the group that travels attentively along, helping and learning at the direction of the dominant figure.

A friend pulls me aside one evening to report an event he claims he has witnessed: An elderly woman in the hospital noticed that the group coming to see her on rounds included a medical student who reminded her of her own beloved grandson. The attending physician was leading the student through an examination of the woman, and had just asked the uncertain student, "What does it look like to you?" A nurse, entering the room with a message for the doctor, distracted him for a moment. Instantly, the patient put a finger to her lips, tugged the medical student close, glanced conspiratorially around, and faintly whispered "Diabetes!" before the doctor turned back to hear the student's confident and correct reply.

One patient may relish all the attention—so many bright, caring people focused intently on one's welfare. Another may resent the duplicated questioning or the repeated probing as one young doctor after another tries to hear the worrying sounds in the lung or feel the abdominal tightness at the place that is painful. A third may even find it an intriguing show, noting how each member of the visiting group has a place in the hierarchy, subtly revealed by patterns of deference and authority. (Who stands in front, who to the rear, when not all can be close enough to see the incision well? Who moves closer at whose invitation? Who feels free to interrupt; who waits for a break in the discussion? Who addresses the patient directly; who responds only to what is said by the attending physician?)

How should I be represented to the patients we will see, I ask. To introduce me as "Dr." would be clearly misleading in this setting. A patient might reasonably object to my being present in an intimate context when I am merely an observer, not part of the health care team. "Mr." is fine with me, I point out. But it raises the question of how to explain what I am doing here. Patient rooms, after all, aren't generally open to tourists. We decide on "Professor," with a brief sentence describing me as a visitor to the hospital who is especially interested in ethical issues in medicine and who is here to observe what goes on. As we make the rounds, no patient objects to my presence, or seems much interested in why I am here. It is enough that I have come in with the doctor.

The issue of how one represents oneself to patients is felt keenly by medical students. In their clinical years, they learn a mass of factual information and develop an assortment of skills, but they typically must apply that knowledge and use those skills without a comfortable command of either. It often seems to them that they are frauds—not yet doctors, but pretending to be, and doing things to patients that the patients might not allow if they fully understood the magnitude of the pretense.

In some teaching hospitals, medical students are introduced to patients by clinical instructors—senior physicians—as "Dr. Smith." In other settings, they are more candidly introduced as "Student Doctor Jones." And sometimes they are frankly described as medical students.

One defense sometimes given for calling these student doctors is the claim that it minimizes patient anxiety and thus contributes to better health care. Another claimed justification is that it accelerates the process of getting the students to think like doctors. In one respect it surely does; it encourages them to see themselves as impostors, and to think of that as a natural part of what their profession allows and at times requires. For the sense of being an impostor often recurs in senior physicians, who know all too well of the uncertainties and limitations of medical practice, and know also that they are often perceived—sometimes with their own complicity—as capable of working miracles.

There is no doubt that medical students feel substantial anxiety about their interactions with patients. They tend to be keenly aware of their lack of experience and, appropriately, deeply uncertain about their capacity to function competently with patients. They readily verbalize their distaste for being misrepresented, and much prefer the increasingly common practice of describing them as the medical students they are.

As medical students, they still live mainly in a world of learning facts, of getting things right or else getting them wrong. Uncertainty is strange and unwelcome to them; they have not yet learned that it will be their constant companion, and they will have to come to terms with the need to base judgments and actions on imperfect information. Indeed, the development, organization, and evaluation of information will emerge as a centrally important part of medical practice.

A friend phones me at the hospital in a state of advanced mirth; he tells me that his brother-in-law, whom I know slightly, has a story about the hospital I must hear. I phone and get the story. Mr. S is a good friend of the hospital. A wealthy man, he has made some generous gifts to it. He has also been a patient, and is grateful to the hospital for saving him from bleeding to death after an assault by a robber some years ago.

Last weekend, he tells me, he twisted his ankle rather badly while working in his yard. His doctor told him to go to the emergency room to have the ankle X rayed. As a former patient, Mr. S had a Beth Israel identification card which he presented to the receptionist on arrival at the emergency room. She typed his name into her computer terminal, looked up at him, and asked, "Mr. S, do you still live at the same address on Williams St.?"

"Yes, I do."

"And you're going to give your organs to the hospital?"
Taken aback, he replied, "Well, yes. But not today. It's only an
injured ankle! What prompted you to ask me that?"
"Oh. Well, it says here on the screen that you're a major donor."

Computerized hospital record systems contain personal information about patients, as do such systems outside the hospital.
The security of these systems is dubious. What distressed the
administrators at Beth Israel when I told them the story of Mr. S
was not the behavior of the receptionist; everyone found that more
amusing than troubling. But information had appeared on her
screen that was never intended to be available to her. The system
had a feature that those who created it and who use it neither
intended it to have nor realized it did have. This is common with
complex systems. We readily create technical systems of various
sorts—Challenger space flights, artificial hearts, and medical
information systems are but cases in point—the complexity of
which we do not and perhaps cannot fully understand.

In designing any information system, it is necessary to make
explicit and reasoned choices about who should have access to
each type of information. A patient's medical record should be
available to that patient's physician. The financial record should
be available to the billing office. Dietary requirements should be
known, daily, in the kitchen. And so on. But no one believes that all
the information about a patient should be available to anyone with
access to a terminal.

When a public figure is hospitalized—perhaps a prominent
athlete, entertainer, or political candidate—there may be substantial public interest in that patient's diagnosis or medical history,
and even a market value to such information. To protect the
confidentiality that every patient is due, a system of access codes is
designed to provide for each inquirer only the information that
person should have. This can go wrong in three ways.

First, the initial judgments about who should have access to
what may be faulty. If access is overly restrictive, people who need
information will not be able to get it efficiently. If access is
underrestricted, confidentiality is compromised.

Second, the system will not be impenetrable. Stories are legion
about precocious teen-aged computer wizards who rapidly break

protective codes of all sorts, often for the sheer joy of meeting the technical challenge rather than for any interest in the information. Concerned about this issue, a colleague once raised it in a course on contemporary moral problems. The following week, a student handed him an envelope containing a list of the names and social security numbers of all students in the class and a printout of the professor's driving record from the state motor vehicle authority. The student had obtained them by telephone, using the computer in his room, as a demonstration of how little protection this information had.

Reflecting the continuing generality of this problem, the *Academic Computing Handbook* published at Syracuse University in 1988 contained this warning:

> You should not expect any password, no matter how elaborate, to absolutely protect electronic information. A good password is like a good door lock: it deters the thief. A determined and clever thief will most likely manage to steal whatever he wants. If you have sensitive information, consider encoding it or keeping it elsewhere than in a mainframe computer. . . .

But the benefits of computerized record systems in hospitals all depend on the information being readily available in plain English, not in code, from a central mainframe computer.

The third problem is the most serious. Any complex software system is almost certain to have features unrealized by its designers. This situation is well described by David Parnas, a widely respected computer scientist with over 20 years of experience in software engineering. Parnas resigned from the Panel on Computing in Support of Battle Management (established as part of President Reagan's Strategic Defense Initiative) in 1985, submitting with his resignation a set of eight short essays explaining "why many computer scientists believe that systems of the sort being considered by the SDIO cannot be built." In the first essay, "Why Software Is Unreliable," he notes that

> The lay public, familiar with only a few incidents of software failure, may regard them as exceptions caused by inept programmers. Those of us who are software professionals know better; the most competent

programmers in the world cannot avoid such problems. . . . Even in highly structured systems, surprises and unreliability occur because the human mind is not able to fully comprehend the many conditions that can arise. . . .

This point is hardly new. Over thirty years ago, I heard Norbert Weiner lecture on the relationship between humans and computing machines; he said, "The more intelligent a machine is, the more it will do what it is told to do. This may differ from what you want it to do. We can give a machine orders which it can carry out before we fully understand the implications of the orders."

Mr. S escaped with his organs intact, and his ankle, which was only sprained, soon healed. So he gained a lovely anecdote from the episode, with no harm done. Still, he had a vivid reminder that one must pay due regard to common sense before acting on the basis of any computer's output. I have met some medical students—just a few—who expressed the hope that computerized information systems will provide a solution to the problems of uncertainty and intellectual fallibility that seem so daunting. That is also a false hope, although computers can provide some limited relief. But they will never substitute for the sensitivity that health care providers must have to their patients.

One patient is from a small town in New England; he has come for an extensive cardiac workup. He is told who I am and why I am present; he greets me deferentially. The Visit is encouraging in speaking to him; although he has some heart problems, they seem manageable. He is in no great danger, and should soon be back at work. But he is greatly agitated about having recently learned that his heart is enlarged. He complains bitterly to the Visit that his own doctor did not explain to him that his cardiomyopathy involved enlargement of the heart. He seems angry; emotionally, he asks, "If my doctor can't confide in me, how can I confide in my doctor?"

The Visit calms him, reassures him. The group moves on, but I drop back, as the patient seems to want to say something to me. "I'm sorry if I sort of lost my temper there. I shouldn't have. But it upsets me."

"There's nothing to apologize for," I tell him. "It's right for you

to express your feelings, including your anger, when you're upset about something here. You know, it even helps your doctors understand better what is going on with you and what is important to you. There's nothing for you to feel sorry about."

He seems relieved. Smiling, he says, "Okay. I understand. That's very helpful. Thank you, Doctor." I catch up with the group, feeling rather like an impostor myself, and continue on the rounds.

Grand rounds is neither grand nor rounds. The phrase is just hospital dialect for a regularly scheduled meeting of a department to hear a lecture or case presentation. Typically, each department will have grand rounds at a set time each week. All the hospital staff associated with that department are expected to attend— senior physicians, house officers, and medical students on that rotation. Others, such as nurses, dieticians, physical therapists, laboratory technicians, may attend according to their interests and schedules. The attending physicians are invited, too, and many of them come as part of their continuing medical education. The topics and speakers are posted in advance, and sometimes attract staff from other departments as well. The subject matter may be the presentation of a current case of particular interest by one of the members of the department, it may be a lecture of more general interest by a specialist from outside the hospital, or it may even be a major, specially funded lecture by a figure of great distinction and renown.

The attendance at medical grand rounds—that is, grand rounds in the department of medicine—is large today. The speaker is a prominent figure from abroad, come to give a series of lectures at various of the medical institutions connected with Harvard Medical School. Most of her lecture washes over me as if in a foreign language, even though it is in the flawless English of a proper British Dame (there is something grand about grand rounds this time). I just don't know enough about portal hypertension to make much sense of this technical exposition. I catch a point here and there—schistosomiasis is the major cause of this problem in some parts of the world; it is an ailment of young men in India, but middle-aged women in Japan. Surgical treatment, I discern, is difficult and unreliable; there is something called a Warren shunt, but it is risky and often unhelpful.

Almost as an aside, the speaker notes softly, "It is often kinder to do nothing at all, but this you can never explain to junior doctors." I sit forward more attentively, eager to follow what comes next. But it was a throwaway line; what follows is all to do with bleeding esophageal varices—with the options, indications, limitations, and uncertainties associated with distal spleno-renal shunts, and the like. Finally, to great applause, the lecture ends and the question period begins.

Most of those in the hall are unknown to me, and I am a stranger to them. I half-listen to a series of technical medical questions and answers, but I am still absorbed by that one remark about the young doctors. There is a lull in the discussion, with a few minutes left in the hour.

I ask, "I am intrigued by your claim that you can never explain to young doctors that it is often kinder to do nothing in such cases. I'd be very interested to know what efforts, what kinds of efforts, you have made to explain it to them, and what you have found the barriers to be that have prevented you from succeeding. Also, I am interested that such an important issue merits just a single sentence. Why is it a less crucial matter than the technical explanation of, say, distal spleno-renal shunts?"

The speaker looks at me in disbelief; she seems to have been blindsided by such a nontechnical question. Her reply starts very wide of the mark: " I can't see what that has to do with the Warren shunt." Then, perhaps realizing that I am asking a question about wisdom, not about skill, she aims with greater care. "The young doctors, they think they will save the patient. I would not want to take that away from them, though if I were to treat the patient without the young doctors I would be less aggressive with the treatment."

The time is nearly up now; in his concluding remarks, the chairman wisely notes, "So much of modern medicine deals with the complications of very complex diseases. If you handle a complication, you may feel very proud, but perhaps you haven't done much for the patient."

As we file out of the hall, the chief of surgery approaches me. "I think she didn't really understand your question," he says. "She *wasn't expecting a question like that, and I think it threw her a bit."* If this was not the proper forum for such a question, I wonder, what is? In the corridor, I overhear two doctors talking earnestly about the question, about how it might have been answered.

.4.

OBGYN

*A*t grand rounds in the department of Obstetrics and Gynecology (OBGYN), the doctors are puzzling together about a case that is being presented clue by clue; the whole discussion has some of the feel of a television game show or a mystery story. The identity of the patient is obscured by changes in the non-essential facts of the case (but a few people know who she is anyway), and the identity of the physician attending the case is kept secret so that the discussion will not be biased by attitudes toward that doctor—who may well be present at the meeting. The point of the exercise is not to make decisions about management of the case, which is already concluded; the discussion is part of the continuing education of the staff and the attending physicians.

The patient is admitted for induction of labor three weeks after her due date. (If a woman is more than two weeks overdue, the situation is considered one of increased risk.) She delivers a large, healthy baby by Cesarean section, but has excessive bleeding and atony of the uterus. (Was the uterus properly massaged prior to closure?) Within half an hour after delivery, she is in unstable condition. A dilation and curettage fails to correct the problem; the uterus is reopened and nothing is found. Her blood figures are falling; drug intervention is to no avail. The physicians responsible for her care make a decision in favor of an emergency hysterectomy. Her blood figures improve, and she is returned to the recovery room. She is given five units of packed red cells, but *her blood pressure won't stabilize. She's bleeding again or is in cardiogenic shock. What to do?*

A senior obstetrician comments on the case. "The people taking care of her are by now knee-deep in anxiety. What she needs at this point is another person, fresh and not involved. Get someone else. Say, 'I've just been through something horrible. Come see if I'm seeing this correctly.'"

We hear more about the case. She stabilizes, but two hours later her blood pressure falls again. An hour later she is back in surgery having various parts resutured. Her severe post-partum hemorrhaging is controlled; she goes home a week later.

Get someone else. Such simple, sound advice—yet it is so often hard to remember in a time of crisis. And, although it is such good advice, it is all too often taken as an affront. (I know of a physician who, when asked some years ago by a patient to arrange a second opinion, did so, but refused thereafter ever to see or speak to that patient again.)

Now, third-party payers increasingly require second opinions as part of the standard process of medical decision making. And the standard codes of medical ethics have long stipulated that a physician must seek consultation when asked to do so or when doing so will enhance the quality of care provided. Yet physicians sometimes refrain from, resist, or resent the simple step of getting someone else. A patient is always entitled to another opinion and a fresh perspective may also be just what the doctor needs, even if it isn't what the doctor ordered. Patients should never be reluctant to assert their right to get someone else, and physicians should be trained to view an independent opinion as an important diagnostic resource.

This is not to say that seeking a second opinion is always unproblematic. Ideally, an independent opinion will lead to new information or understanding that clarifies, without disagreement, what ought to be done. If the second opinion differs substantially from the first, however, it becomes necessary to adjudicate the difference somehow. That can go well, as the sources of the opinions confer about the case. But it can also lead to a standoff, requiring either a third opinion or a forced choice between two irreconcilable points of view. If the patient is competent and kept informed of the deliberations about the case, learning of such uncertainty among physicians about how to proceed can be a cause of great confusion, distress, and loss of confidence. And additional opinions increase costs. So the point is not that, in general, more opinions are better, but only that one should always be open to the possibility that another opinion is exactly what is needed. Opinions may differ, of course, about just when another opinion should be sought.

At another grand rounds in OBGYN the discussion is about ovulation, gametogenesis, and implantation. The hospital has an in vitro *fertilization clinic; childless couples come with the hope that modern medical technology can overcome their infertility. The clinic has not had to face the issue of requests for service from unmarried couples or single women, since Massachusetts law restricts its availability to married couples only. The hospital receives such requests, but dismisses them automatically, citing state law. The couples accepted into the program suffer from blocked Fallopian tubes, oligospermic cervical factor, or two years of unexplained infertility. Ideally, four embryos result from the* in vitro *fertilization, and all are implanted. There is a small risk of multiple births, but the most common outcome is a lack of success in establishing a pregnancy at all.*

I am surprised to learn that "conception in the watchglass" was discussed in the medical literature nearly fifty years ago. But the procedure has only been successful as a clinical therapy since 1978, when Louise Brown was born in England. It works well, leading to normal pregnancies and births, when it works. But it only works a small percentage of the time. I start to learn why.

The fertilization life of an ovum is 12 to 24 hours, and capacitation of the sperm requires several hours in a female environment. The sperm, entering the ovum, fertilizes it through a process that occurs over time, giving the lie to any notion of "the instant of conception." Understood at the microscopic level, conception is a slow unfolding of many events.

Fertilization occurs fairly easily in vitro, *as it does* in vivo. *The real challenge comes later with implantation. That, too, is a complex process with many stages. Failure of implantation accounts for the greatest loss of embryos both with natural and* in vitro *fertilization. The alignment can be wrong; the embryo can implant in inappropriate places. There can be immunological aspects of the process, the biochemistry of which is not well known. Some metastatic processes have analogous aspects.*

The discussion centers on the mysteries of implantation—on the great uncertainty about the difference between when it works and when it doesn't. I ask if progress in this area of medicine has been impeded by the federal moratorium (in effect for nearly a decade) against support for research involving IVF. My question surprises one of the doctors. "I thought you were going to ask when life begins," he notes with relief. He adds that, of course, the moratorium has been a great hindrance to medical progress.

The moratorium was adopted by the then Department of Health, Education and Welfare in the late 1970s, when a research proposal to the National Institutes of Health raised the question of the ethical justifiability of research involving *in vitro* fertilization of humans. The question was studied at length by a departmental Ethics Advisory Board comprising scientists, various clergymen, and many others. After holding open hearings in every region of the country, the Board determined that such research is entirely appropriate under limited circumstances, and recommended that the moratorium be lifted.

That moratorium has no scientific support, and the government's own inquiry determined that it has no legitimate basis in social policy. But a small, vocal, organized constituency opposes IVF, and the matter is politically sensitive. So no government official with the authority to do so has had the courage to lift the moratorium. Much of the opposition to lifting the moratorium was systematically orchestrated by the anti-abortion or "Right to Life" movement, which opposed the clinical use of *in vitro* fertilization on various grounds—for example, that some embryos might be unused and therefore discarded or abused, that technologically assisted human reproduction is unnatural and therefore wrong, or that further development of such technology would likely lead to unacceptable applications. What an irony that couples whose fondest hope is to have a child of their own, and who are typically motivated by thoroughly traditional and genuinely pro-life family values, are most vigorously opposed by a constituency that marches under the banner of those same values! The Ethics Advisory Board has long since been disbanded, even though the regulations of the Department of Health and Human Services require that such a board exist. The original Board's report has gone unanswered for a decade. Today, IVF is the only widely available clinical therapy that cannot be studied in any federally operated facility or federally supported program.

Over one hundred centers in this country now provide IVF. No reason has emerged to think the procedure is unsafe. But it is expensive and often fails. Indeed, many centers have yet to achieve their first successful outcome. A better understanding of why *in vitro* fertilization fails would be much more likely if this area of research were treated like all others, with research proposals supported if they satisfy the two criteria of having high scientific merit and surviving systematic ethical scrutiny. And that understanding would not only benefit potential IVF recipients, it would also shed light on correctable barriers to natural reproduction—and possibly on immunological and metastatic processes, as well. But even satisfying both of these criteria is not enough in the case of research related to IVF. Thus can the heavy hand of political cowardice stifle the quest for greater understanding of fundamental biological processes.

I sit in my office reading. An obstetrician phones to ask me to speak at grand rounds. I gladly agree, pleased by the request in part because OBGYN, despite the problems it confronts, also seems to be the happiest unit of the hospital. I've been hanging around intensive care units all day, where nobody looks good. The patients are in serious condition, often unable to communicate much, and the staff show the strain on their faces and in their hushed tones. It will be a treat to do some more business with a jollier crowd.

A sense of optimism and satisfaction is abundant on the labor and delivery unit. There are problems here, to be sure. There is a high-risk pregnancy program, with attendant challenges for the staff, fears for the patients, and occasional disappointments for both. Tragedy does occur, including stillborn or seriously damaged children. There is no Level I neonatal intensive care unit at the hospital, however, so the very sickest infants are immediately transferred to a nearby facility. From time to time there is a gravely ill patient, like the woman with post-partum hemorrhaging.

A 71-year-old woman has ovarian cancer that has spread. The ingredients of treatment are surgery, chemotherapy, radiation, and withholding aggressive treatment in favor of providing comfort care only. What the case management should be varies with the "geography" of the lesions. Following initial surgery, this woman has had whole abdomen radiation therapy without chemotherapy. She has now deteriorated seriously; gravely ill, she is in the medical intensive care unit, almost totally unresponsive. One gynecologist complains, "The neurologists feel it's a minor event, that she should recover!" The woman's two daughters want "everything possible to be done as long as there is any uncertainty," he continues. "But her goose was cooked as soon as you found at surgery that the disease had spread. It's a no-win situation."

Another woman, in her eighth month of pregnancy, is basically healthy, but it has recently come to light that she is a heroin user. If her use is occasional, she is at great risk for an overdose, and the treatment for heroin overdose is likely to lead to fetal damage or even death. If the woman is an addict, her risk of overdose is lower; putting her on a methadone treatment regimen will lower the risk of infection, and likely improve her nutrition and prenatal care. But withdrawal from methadone is slow for infants, taking two to three months. Not a happy start for a youngster. So social and psychological approaches, with monitoring, may be better, especially if she is not an addict.

The case must be reported if there is evidence of fetal symptoms, but not simply because the woman is known to use illegal drugs. I picture some poor, uneducated woman, living amidst the drug culture in ignorance and squalor. How can she be made to understand, I wonder. How can her behavior be influenced? "There's one more thing," the doctor presenting the case points out. "This woman is in the medical profession herself."

The doctors and nurses gathered to discuss Cesarean sections agree that the procedure is over-used, and that the fact that a woman has had one delivery by C-section is no reason for subsequent deliveries to be by C-section. But many cases are complicated, and it is often very difficult to know how much risk to accept before calling for surgical delivery. One woman is diabetic; shoulder dysplasia places her fetus at risk, so elective C-section is suggested by the case. Another woman delivered a very small baby who looked fine for about four hours, before rapidly going into a fatal decline.

The discussion, somber and unhurried, turns to the problem of strep infections. A young obstetrician reports on his survey of the literature. "I read about sixty papers on the subject. The literature is full of controversy. About half the newborns with strep die from the infection. The disease is treatable in the mothers; the problem is with the babies. It is very fulminant in babies. The infants pick it up during delivery from vaginal infection. That's why we sometimes use antibiotics so liberally. The question is, with a febrile mother, when do we bail out?" A lengthy debate ensues about where to draw the line between avoiding risks of surgery and honoring the preference for vaginal delivery on the one hand, and using surgery to reduce risk on the other hand. The conclusion is that a C-section is justified in the case of a strep-infected woman who cannot be cleared of the infection before delivery.

Despite such problems, mostly this is a cheerful place. Elsewhere one has an inescapable awareness of illness, struggle, and uncertainty. Patients get better, to be sure, but there isn't much visible evidence of it in the hospital. Most in-patients, at least a substantial part of the time, emanate waves of discomfort, anxiety, and dysfunction. As they recover, their focus is typically on getting out, on going home. The hospital shares that focus, so as soon as a patient is securely on the mend, discharge follows quickly. No more lounging around for an extra few days, feeling better and better, gaining strength, chatting up the staff with increasing good humor. That went out with the days when a hospital was paid more if a patient stayed longer.

Now, the payment a hospital receives for each patient depends primarily on the diagnosis—a fixed sum, based on the patient's diagnosis related group (DRG). So it makes good economic sense for the hospital to send them home sooner—even if sicker—as long as they seem safely headed toward recovery. Early reports indicate that the system seems to be working. Hospital stays have become shorter, but the rates of recovery from illness do not seem to have suffered as a result—although there is as yet no conclusive judgment about the effect on quality of care. Yet there is a cost that is taking its toll in hospitals.

Patients may be just as likely to regain good health in the end, but since the staff sees less of that recovery, there's less gratification in providing health care. There just isn't the sense of visible success that once was there to spur health care providers on and to sustain them through the tougher aspects of their work. There is some satisfaction in knowing that a patient is improving, and in sending her home confident that she will soon feel entirely well. But it isn't the same as seeing that payoff unfold before one's eyes. The result is one more turn of the dehumanizing screws in medical practice.

But the pregnant patients typically aren't hoping to be made well again. They're not looking for relief from illness or injury. Theirs is a climate of enthusiasm and discovery. Most of them will have healthy new babies, and the staff will see and share in their excitement and joy. Most patients will leave with a sense of being better off than they were before, not merely hoping to recover to their previous state. Despite the disappointments and even tragedies that spoil the party from time to time, the basic tone of the place is definitely upbeat.

My caller is raising the question of a topic. It should be no problem; there are so many issues we could discuss. I mention one of them—the problem of developing an ethically appropriate set of policies toward the use of in vitro *fertilization, frozen embryo transfer, egg donation, and other aspects of technologically aided human reproduction. I'm sure he'll be pleased at the suggestion. Having an IVF program, the hospital won't be able to avoid coming to terms with some of the other issues in high-tech reproduction as consumers demand more sophisticated treatments for infertility, and as other hospitals develop more sophisticated responses. Or, we could discuss the issues surrounding surrogate motherhood.*

"Yes," I hear him say, "these are all important problems that we must worry about one day. But perhaps it would be more useful for us to hear your thoughts about what worries us now. I think what we would appreciate most would be for you to talk to us about abortion."

I am aghast. Of all the tired, boring, overdiscussed issues, this is the last one I expected to be asked to speak about. It is certainly the last one I am motivated to speak about. One could make a career of reading what has already been written on the subject, or of cataloguing the varieties of bad arguments and bad manners on all sides of the endless debate. And once one had done it all, it is unlikely that anything intellectually new or socially useful would emerge as a result. But it is what they want. Hiding my disappointment as well as I can, I agree to discuss, yet again, The Problem of Abortion. But I wonder if I have anything to say that will be worth hearing.

I turn to the file I have been keeping of recent newspaper and magazine clippings, mainly from the Boston Globe, about intriguing issues in health care. They appear every few days, so even though I have been in town only briefly, the file has grown fat. A man whose foot was severed in a mowing accident has had it reattached. A comotose man's guardian opposes the removal of his feeding tube. Another man's wife petitions the court to have his feeding tube removed. The Massachusetts Medical Society adopts a policy allowing for the removal of feeding tubes. Layoffs at Concord Hospital reflect a drop in hospital use; the trend is showing up all over the country. An advertisement in Boston magazine seeks a woman to be a surrogate mother. Respondents are to write to an unnamed law firm at a post office box, enclosing information and a picture; the successful applicant will be paid a surrogacy fee of $50,000.

"Fetal viability overlaps legal abortion line" reads the headline of one article. Advances in the care of very premature infants have now made it possible, on rare occasions, to save the lives of infants born, to everyone's surprise, as a result of an attempted abortion that has succeeded in terminating a pregnancy, but without resulting in fetal death. I've heard of four such cases in all; two lived but briefly, one achieved good health, and one survived as a very severely damaged and permanently handicapped child.

I sit looking at the headline, aware that I've agreed to talk about abortion, realizing for the first time that I don't even know what an abortion is anymore. All that rancorous, oversimplified debate about abortion rights seems to assume that there is a common understanding of what is in dispute. But if a woman has a right to an abortion, what is it she has a right to do?

Is it just a right to have her pregnancy terminated, or is it also a right to assurance that no live birth will occur as a result—a right not to become the parent of an unwanted child? If some methods of abortion allow for the possibility of a live fetus and others do not, does a right to an abortion require the right to determine the method that will be used? It seems to me that it must, but that is a substantial revision of current understandings.

They want to hear my thoughts on abortion, but I may be accused of making matters worse, not better.

Professional staff within the hospital know that what they do can affect and be affected by the larger surrounding communities. A zealous and politically ambitious public prosecutor, for example, can seize on a medical episode in a thoroughly disruptive way. Or the press can create substantial turmoil within and about a hospital if it covers a controversial matter in even a slightly sensationalistic way. Since the traditions of Catholic thought that dominate Boston's political life are different in some respects from the traditions of thought that are most evident within the hospital, it makes particularly good sense for staff in the hospital to be sensitive to their larger community.

The "Baby Doe" episode served well to accentuate the sense within the medical world that the smart doctor these days must keep one eye on the door at all times. Reacting to a now famous case on Long Island, in which a question was raised about whether a handicapped infant would receive appropriate treatment, the Department of Health and Human Services established a policy requiring all federally funded hospitals to post notices of a toll-free "hotline" that would receive calls, including anonymous tips, to the effect that a handicapped infant was being denied proper care because of the handicap. Federal investigators could then be dispatched to the scene to see that justice was done.

That infamous Baby Doe Hotline was short lived; a federal court found that the administration had acted capriciously and without due regard to proper procedure in establishing it. New policies, fashioned in part as a result of negotiation with medical organizations as well as with advocates of the rights and interests of the handicapped, are less onerous. (And the Supreme Court has now held that the sort of neonatal crises at issue are not the government's proper business.) But the medical world remembers those notices and that hotline, and knows that any disgruntled person, with good evidence, bad evidence, or none, can call a newspaper or district attorney and thereby cause at least a costly distraction.

Curious about how the Baby Doe Hotline was working, I had called it in April 1983. I was told that the line could only be used to report cases of suspected abuse, but that if I left my name and number, someone would return the call who could answer my questions. Within minutes, a member of the HHS staff did return the call. I learned that the hotline had received at that point about 500 calls. Most of them were about tax questions, veterans' benefits, social security, the national parks, and other matters unrelated to the purpose of the hotline. A free line to Washington, it seems, has broad appeal.

Only a handful of calls reported complaints of the appropriate type, and some of those were quickly found to be hoaxes. In four cases, the Department was able to confirm that the caller was lodging a serious complaint about a real infant. In at least one of those cases—but possibly just one—a neonatal intensive care unit was disrupted by the sudden arrival of a squad of federal marshalls and local police. In the end, nothing inappropriate was found to have been happening in respect to the treatment of the infant. But the fact that the disruption occurred at all quickly emphasized in nursery units across the land that malpractice suits are not the only peril hanging over the heads of neonatologists.

One mistreated infant would be one too many; preventing one such abuse is an objective that must command respect. But one disrupted hospital unit is also a lot, for it is enough to demonstrate the reality of direct government involvement in particular patient care decisions, even where there is complete agreement among family and medical team members about what ought to be done.

That's a demonstration that health care providers don't need to see many times to develop a sense of caution about how what they do will be perceived by outsiders.

A member of the hospital's Ethics Committee stops me in the corridor. He is concerned about a request that has come to the hospital from a medical scientist at a nearby hospital, who is doing research that requires the use of fetal tissue. He has asked that Beth Israel allow him access to the fetal material that becomes available here. Is it a good idea, I am asked, to agree to provide that material to him?

There is great sensitivity about the request. The research protocol is solid; it adheres to the federal guidelines governing research on fetal material and it holds reasonable promise of adding usefully to the sum of medical understanding. And, like nearly hospitals, Beth Israel has a certain amount of fetal material available.

I recall that the research leading to a vaccine for Rubella, which earned a Nobel Prize, was done in Scandinavia rather than in the United States because it depended on the use of fetal tissue. There is no reason to oppose fetal research on ethical grounds, I point out, provided it satisfies the various relevant guidelines. But the question before us sounds as though it is less an ethical question than a political one. Perhaps it would be imprudent for this hospital, considering its larger political environment, to invite the attention of the critics of fetal research by assisting such a project elsewhere, even if it is a worthy project. The opponents of a particular type of research can often gain the willing ear of the media and create significant distraction, if not disruption, even without noting fine distinctions or paying much regard to the merits of a case.

Later, I learn that, after serious debate and reflection on the part of many staff members, the hospital has decided to decline the request in light of sensitivities and controversy in the surrounding community about the legitimacy of such research.

More recently, public and governmental attention has focused on the experimental use of fetal tissue in therapy for such diseases as Parkinson's and diabetes. There is some evidence, as yet inconclusive, that the implantation of fetal tissue may have beneficial therapeutic effect.

Because of the distinctive physical characteristics of fetal tissue, there is no substitute for its use. And, because fetal tissue is frequently available as a by-product of natural processes that occur without deliberate intervention, it will always continue to be available.

To prevent the doing of good is as wrong as to do harm; indeed, it is to do a kind of harm. Can there be any respectable argument against the further medical use of fetal tissue? Is there any justification for opposing or impeding that use?

Two facts at least are clear: (1) there is strong therapeutic and investigative reason to continue, and (2) there is deeply entrenched opposition to the practice. That opposition comes from many quarters of very different character.

Some of the opponents are among those whose judgments are driven by a naive passion for simplicity. When they perceive dangers to be associated with something, they need know nothing more in order to be against it, no matter how scant or unlikely the dangers and no matter how great the benefits that stand to be lost. There are some dangers associated with the medical use of fetal tissue—as there are with nearly everything else of any complexity—and this provides them with the basis for their resistance.

Another source of opposition comes from those whose capacity to reason shuts down when they hear the word "fetus." They, too, thrive on oversimplification, and acknowledge no distinctions among the various categories of activity under debate. In particular, they equate fetal tissue with living fetuses, and object to doing with one what would be clearly wrong to do with the other, despite the obvious differences.

These two kinds of opposition have provided much of the energy and political influence that have impeded both medical progress and sound public policy determination in the United States in recent years. But they are not the whole story, for there are also some grounds for concern that will bear scrutiny.

Fetal tissue, because of what it is, is not a mere pharmaceutical commodity. Its origin is in living human beings; for that reason precisely, it is medically valuable. And for that reason, as well, we must be seriously concerned both about how it is obtained and about the network of social practices that surround its use.

Because its proper use can improve and save lives, the imperative of beneficence creates a powerful pressure to use it. Then what is there to fear?

Whatever the limits are on the justifiability of abortion, it would be wrong for women to become pregnant and then abort for the purpose of producing, as a marketable commodity, fetal tissues. Just as it is wrong to use persons as means only, rather than respecting them as ends unto themselves, it is wrong also to use human beings that way, even if they are not yet fully persons.

The corrective to this and related risks is not to ban the use of fetal tissue, however. It is to do as we have done in the case of human kidneys, by prohibiting a commercial market in the tissues in question. If there is no market value to fetal tissues, they will not be brought to market, despite their value for humane purposes.

It would also be wrong to view any fetus—whether it is the result of spontaneous or induced abortion makes no difference—as simply a source of tissue, without due consideration of its stage of development, of whether it is living or dead, and of the attitude of the woman whose issue it is. But the remedy is not to ban the use of fetal tissue, any more than we ban the use of cadaver tissue. The remedy is to regulate that use sensitively and intelligently, making the distinctions that make the difference before reaching decisions about what should be done.

We take cadaver organs and transplant them; we use human bodies for medical instruction; we perform autopsies to learn more about disease processes. In doing these things, we have lost no respect for human life or for persons. On the contrary, it is because of our fundamental regard for life and for the wellbeing of humankind that we do such otherwise distasteful things. We do not do them capriciously, arbitrarily, or without appropriate consent.

The same attitude should govern our use of fetal tissues. We should not scorn those who point to the possible excesses that lie ahead. It is necessary instead to construct safeguards that effectively exclude those excesses. But neither should we allow public policy to be dominated by the pressures of those who would crudely and cruelly ignore crucial distinctions and simplistically oppose whatever makes them uneasy. There is too much at stake, in human life and human health, for that.

In 1988, the Director of the National Institutes of Health constituted the Human Fetal Tissue Transplantation Research Panel as an ad hoc consultants' group to the Advisory Committee to the Director. The Panel was charged to review the "ethical, legal, and scientific issues surrounding the use of human fetal tissue derived from induced abortions in transplantation research." After a broad-based and open inquiry, that highly prestigious Panel concluded that the moratorium then in effect on federal support for such research should be lifted. The Panel submitted its report to the Advisory Committee, including dissenting minority opinions. In December 1988, the Advisory Committee unanimously recommended the acceptance of the Panel's report and the lifting of the moratorium. Once again, however, history seems to have been repeated. An ideological administration has ignored the conclusions of the inquiry it commissioned because the results were politically displeasing, and the moratorium, as of early 1990, remains in effect.

At Boston's Beth Israel, a large turnout at grand rounds confirmed substantial interest in the topic of my lecture on abortion. It had become clear to me, on the basis of several conversations with others in the hospital, that the interest had diverse origins. The members of the hospital community were sensitive to the various issues surrounding abortion, but had differing interpretations of the most serious difficulties related to abortion. Most of those I talked with seemed to have a cautious pro-choice position; that is, they were in favor of abortion's being available as an option in a variety of circumstances, but viewed it as a serious, unfortunate step that should not ever be viewed as trivial. And most seemed genuinely confused by the apparent overlap between the earliest weeks of viability and the latest weeks of access to abortion. Some, in addition, were concerned that unless the advocates of choice actively accepted some limitation in response to that overlap, there might be a repressive reaction that would seriously reduce access even in the early weeks for women who had powerful reasons to make the unhappy choice to abort.

I knew that I must disappoint any who came hoping for an answer to "the problem of abortion," whatever they took that problem to be. But perhaps it would be useful for them to hear my thoughts about why no such answer can reasonably be expected. Those thoughts follow.

It is a confusion to think there are simply two opposing camps— the "pro-life" and the "pro-choice" teams. That confusion is natural enough in a climate of public debate that seems to demand that the battle lines be drawn with increasing clarity. But the strongest advocates of both "pro-life" and "pro-choice" positions seem like cartoon characters in their stridency and insensitivity to the opposition's motivation. For most people, the issues are just not so clear; some instances of abortion seem justified and others not. What typically divides people is not whether they are simply for or against abortion, but how they draw the line between these two categories.

In an excellent opinion piece in *Newsweek* (March 25, 1985), Rachel Richardson Smith describes herself as being "in the awkward position of being both anti-abortion and pro-choice." She objects that these two camps fail to "recognize the grey area where I seem to be languishing" and she notes that "no woman wants to have an abortion. Circumstances demand it; women do it." But never with joy. "Relief, yes. But also ambivalence, grief, despair, guilt." Smith then asks of abortion decisions, "Why is it not akin to the same painful experience families must sometimes make to allow a loved one to die? . . . How can we change the context in which we think about abortion?"

The old context is one of extreme positions. One example is that of Michael Tooley, a philosopher whose writing has reached a broad nonacademic audience. He argues that "An organism possesses a serious right to life only if it possesses the concept of a self as a continuing subject of experience . . . and believes that it is itself such a continuing entity." Since the fetus at every stage lacks any such concept or belief, there is no right to life to protect, even in very late stage abortions. Indeed, Tooley recognizes, and welcomes, the conclusion that since the newborn infant lacks the concept of a continuing self, "infanticide during a period shortly after birth must be morally acceptable."* He suggests selecting a modest period of time—a week after birth—during which the desirability of infanticide may be assessed; in this way, he claims,

* "Abortion and Infanticide," *Philosophy and Public Affairs* 2:1, 1972.

"The practical moral problem can thus be satisfactorily handled."
A consequence of this position is that it is permissible to kill a
newborn child who is discovered at birth to have a horrible
developmental disorder, just as it is permissible to abort an early
term fetus to prevent the birth of a child with that same disorder.

An equally extreme position appears in *Health Care Ethics*,
published in 1982 by the Catholic Health Care Association of the
United States. After identifying nine "considerations frequently
cited in favor of a woman's right to make this decision," the
authors (Ashley and O'Rourke) conclude that "The advantages for
the woman and for society are very tangible and in a concrete
situation many may concur and the opposite disadvantages of
pregnancy seem so overwhelming, especially if the woman is poor,
already heavily burdened with children, and physically or psychologically ill, that she may very well believe that there is no other
way out. . . . Faced with a woman in such a dilemma, any
compassionate health care professional may also believe that it
would be utterly cruel and inhumane to refuse the medical
cooperation she requests."

There are, however, seven considerations of varying degrees of
persuasiveness offered on the other side of the issue. (For example, no. 4: "Abortion policies tend to exclude the father from his
proper responsibility for pregnancy and for the child and from his
role of supporting his wife and sharing her burdens. Hence, he,
too, is degraded as a person and burdened with deep conflicts.")
The question then is how to balance "so many positive and
negative consequences of abortion one against another" so as to
reach a conclusion. But the answer, it turns out, is easy, because
the cumulative weight of the positive considerations can never be
equal to "the one basic value of that person's right to live"—where
"that person" is the fetus in question. Since whatever the advantages of an abortion may be to a pregnant woman, it "dooms the
child irretrievably," the prohibition against it must be unyielding.
Thus, "authoritative Catholic documents consistently support the
moral rule that direct killing of innocent human beings can never
be ethically justifiable."

Here we have an assortment of terms used to refer to the fetus:
"child," "person," and "human being." By designating the fetus as
a person, without argument or support for doing so, the authors set

the stage for their ready dismissal of an abortion's benefits for the pregnant woman, no matter how great. For, the argument goes, when a child's life is at issue, no benefits to the woman can outweigh the value of that life. The problem here, however, not even acknowledged by Ashley and O'Rourke, is simply that we do not all agree that an embryo or early stage fetus should count as a child in the first place. And to assume that it should is to beg the question at issue, guaranteeing that one's reasoning will lead to the conclusion that has been accepted all along—that abortion is never justifiable.

These authors refer explicitly to Tooley's position, so they must know that he has discussed the significance of how the terms "person," "fetus," and "human being" are used in these arguments. Nonetheless, they call the fetus a person or child throughout, rather than using morally neutral language—not, I trust, to be deceptive in argument, but because they thoroughly believe that their use of language is accurate.

I do not believe that it makes sense to count an embryo or early term fetus as being a child or person (as I have argued elsewhere; see, for example, *Doctors' Dilemmas,* Chapter 10, "Progeny, Progress, and Primrose Paths"). Instead, I believe it more reasonable to think of personhood and status as a child as properties that a fetus gradually acquires over time, just as it acquires the neurological structure that is necessary for consciousness, a sense of self, and a relationship with others. How, then, am I to judge the opinions and arguments of those who believe as a matter of basic commitment that inviolable personhood is present from the time of conception?

I have no inclination to see them as intolerant fools or austere moralists devoid of human sensitivity, any more than I see Tooley as callously sanctioning the murder of innocents. I do see them both as starkly etched exemplars of opposing camps, each of whose position is unpalatable to most of us between.

Smith shows us how one individual can internalize parts of the outlooks of such opposing camps with incompatible views; the result is an internalized conflict that makes the issue a highly stressful one. There is nothing inconsistent in such an attitude, no more than in any other context in which we are at once attracted to and repelled by something that offers a benefit to us at a distasteful cost. That ambivalence about abortion is widespread, and we ought never to lose sight of it in the continuing public debate. But why is that debate so very difficult to resolve?

Sometimes in setting public policy, after all the economic, legal, and political analysis is in, moral conflict remains a barrier to a resolution of the policy question. Nonetheless, in some of these cases, careful assessment of the value issues in dispute and of the arguments surrounding them leads to a stable, broadly accepted decision. In other cases, no such happy result is attainable, and the dispute lingers on, sustaining bitter social divisiveness. What accounts for the difference between these two kinds of outcome?

We can approach this question by contrasting two examples of policy determination, one of each kind. The lingering case is that of abortion policy; the case that has been satisfactorily resolved concerns a commercial market in transplantable kidneys. Before addressing the cases directly, it is useful to consider a general feature of our structures of belief and value.

We all have some false beliefs as well as some true ones. (The trick is to tell them apart.) Recent work in cognitive psychology teaches us much about how our beliefs are formed—about how we make judgments—and demonstrates that the evidence available to us is only one of many factors that influence what we think is true.

Consider the proposition that when you turn the next page of this book you will find a paid advertisement for a pornographic video cassette. Almost certainly, you think that proposition is false. Your judgment is based on a cluster of beliefs about Oxford University Press in particular and about how publishers and authors address their financial needs in general. Yet we can readily describe evidence that would cause you to give up your belief that no such advertisement is here.

If you turn the page and see one, you will change your mind. That change of mind will cost you something. With puzzlement and disappointment you will realize that the book, author, and publisher are not quite what you thought. Still, that disappointment will not prevent you from giving up your belief that there is no such ad. (The example is not as thoroughly farfetched as it may seem. Dr. Benjamin Spock once found to his dismay that advertisements for various child care products were bound into some editions of his classic *Baby and Child Care*. It took prodigious effort on his part to put an end to that situation, which had occurred without his prior knowledge or consent.)

Compare this with your belief that the person you trust and admire most—spouse, parent, or friend—is innocent of a recent, shocking charge of participating in an organized ring involving drug distribution, extortion, and murder. On hearing the charge, you will likely dismiss it as ludicrous. As the evidence builds, leading to indictment, you may still strongly believe that the charge is false—perhaps based on misunderstandings, coincidences, and misperceptions. And when at the trial you are overwhelmed by the direct evidence, by the videotapes and all the rest, you relinquish your trust at immense personal cost. You will not merely have lost a trusted friend or relative, you will have lost the belief that you have the capacity to judge others and hence to feel secure in your relationships with others. That is a central, crucially important belief; giving it up is emotionally devastating, and that is a large part of why your resistance to the accumulating evidence was so great.

Yet some beliefs are even more centrally imbedded in our way of viewing the world—so thoroughly entrenched in our structures of belief that it is impossible to imagine *any* evidence that would make us give them up. That is the nature of our beliefs, for example, that ten is greater than five, or that what is entailed by true premises must itself be true. We cannot give them up because we literally cannot make any sense of the idea of their being false. They are among our most deeply fundamental beliefs.

So it is with our values. Just as some beliefs are peripheral to our capacity to understand and live in the world, so that we can give them up on the basis of relatively little evidence, some of our values are peripheral to our sense of who and what we are, and how we fit into the world of human interaction. Others are fundamental values that we will not give up no matter what pressure is brought to bear on us to do so. And that is the key point in understanding why some policy disputes are resolvable and others are intractable.

The proposal to allow a commercial market in kidneys had a *prima facie* plausibility. Its advocates argued that if a very poor person who was healthy sold one kidney to an affluent dialysis patient waiting for a transplant, everyone would benefit. The seller would be released from the bonds of poverty, the buyer's medical circumstances would improve, and the organ shortage would be reduced. If the transaction were well informed and fully voluntary, it would be, in economists' terms, Pareto optimal—that is, some or all parties would benefit and no one would be harmed. It would be immoral, the advocates claimed, to deny people the freedom to participate voluntarily in such exchanges. Yet many critics had moral qualms about the plan.

In the debate that followed, critics of the scheme successfully argued that the most desirable societal response to the desperation of poverty and of grave illness is compassion and cooperation, rather than commerce. By the end of Congressional debate on the issue, a consensus had been reached that we do not wish to be the kind of society in which it can make sense for individuals to sell their organs to others; we prefer to continue to work toward solutions to grave economic and medical problems that are driven by a sense of community and mutual concern, rather than by desperation or by market forces.

This consensus was achievable, on the basis of essentially moral arguments, because no substantial constituency was threatened in its fundamental values by the resolution of the debate. Even staunch defenders of the free market have always acknowledged that at least some goods—material as well as social—cannot justifiably be distributed purely by unconstrained market mechanisms. And the advocates of kidney patients have never held that every possible means of increasing the supply of organs is defensible, however rooted it might be in deception or coercion. Nobody's basic view of the world was at stake in this debate.

Just the opposite is true in the debate about abortion policy. There is no more centrally entrenched value than a person's sense of what it is to be a member of the human community. To yield on that kind of point is to lose one's grip on how one ought to live one's life and on how the structures of social organization should function. For those who see the developing fetus as a person in the making, whose moral status evolves gradually as it develops the physiological structures that allow for cognition and sentience, a policy that gives primacy to reproductive autonomy makes the most sense. That is not to say that abortion is to be taken lightly or to deny the presence of strong ambivalence about abortion; it is to say only that in a substantial range of cases, it can be viewed as the least bad alternative.

For those who see the fetus as endowed from the outset with personhood or full moral standing, such a view makes much less sense. For each of these two constituencies, their view of the status of the fetus is not a matter of scientific fact, but of metaphysical commitment. It is a function of beliefs about the nature of the moral order, about what it is to be a person and what kinds of obligations we have toward one another.

That is why every attempt in Congress to resolve the conflict about abortion by means of a "human life amendment" is fatally flawed. Such efforts seek to end dispute by having Congress enact a bill affirming that human life begins at conception. But any such effort, at least on reflection, is ludicrous. No one has ever seriously doubted the fact that the human embryo and fetus are instances of human life. That the human conceptus is human is trivially true. Women do not seek embryo implantations in order to give birth to pandas or parrots, nor do they seek abortions out of fear of delivering koalas or Komodo dragons. If it is alive, it is obviously an instance of human life. And if it were not alive, no question of implantation or of abortion would arise. So the claim is true that, from the time of conception (insofar as the notion makes sense), there is human life at stake, but it is true in a thoroughly uninteresting way that has no bearing on the debate about either what should be permitted as a response to infertility or what should be permitted under abortion policy.

Asserting such an obvious fact—or even discovering an obscure one—cannot resolve these conflicts, because the conflicts are not over matters of fact. They arise out of a clash between different, incompatible ways of viewing the world of human development and interaction. That is a clash of fundamental values, not resolvable in any straightforward way.

Nor is the relationship between reproductive autonomy and the legitimate powers of the state a peripheral issue; it is linked to deeply felt commitments about what it is to be an individual and what a government is for. We do not easily yield on such matters, especially as they are largely immune to influence by evidence.

Our society is pluralistic; in that fact lies much of its splendor and much of its strife. We are condemned to live with an unend-ingly rancorous debate about abortion because the deeply en-trenched values of some large constituency are rejected by each possible policy. The 1989 Supreme Court decision in the Webster case affirms the right of states to enact legislation that, to an as yet untested extent, can restrict access to abortion. The one clear result of that decision will be legislative chaos. States have already begun to differ in their responses. The country will become a patchwork of divergent policies, making access to abortion a function of ability to afford to travel easily; legislators will become increasingly the target of single-issue interest groups on both sides; and the national discord over abortion policy will be aug-mented by the cacophony of discord within the states. But that will be no fundamental change in the basic reality, which is that many people will continue fervently to oppose the availability of abor-tions even as many others fight to secure it; women will continue, one way or another, to have them; and whatever public policy results will be as unstable as that which was in effect between *Roe* v. *Wade* and Webster. Even if *Roe* v. *Wade* is overturned, the instability will persist. The greatest loss may not even be in access to abortion, except perhaps for the poor. It may be in the quality of public policy formation generally, as capable, dedicated people are increasingly discouraged from entering public service—or are run out of it—by anti-abortion groups or pro-choice groups for whom that single issue is of such fundamental importance as to domi-nate political choice.

Yet we do achieve a congenial resolution of some issues that seem at first to bedevil us with moral dispute. In each such case, it is important to go beyond the recognition that moral controversy is impeding the progress of policy determination and to discover the nature and origins of that controversy. Only with a clear idea of the centrality of the value issues in dispute can we also be clear about the prospects for resolution.

Such controversies arise across the spectrum of public policy debates; they are not limited to matters related to health. For example, is manned space exploration worth the human cost? Do the advantages of increasing reliance on chemical products jus-tify the risks of their production and use? If we apply stringent standards of environmental protection, are we unfair to those whose jobs are threatened? Is capital punishment ever justifiable in a civilized society? The list of such policy questions goes on and on—questions that leave us, after all the available facts are gathered, to face the uncertainty of what is right to do.

These questions will increasingly dominate the agendas of policy debate, and have already become central in the setting of health policy. Should we ever limit on economic grounds what we spend on medical care for the extremely old? Is it justifiable to make quality of life assessments for patients whose lives we can sustain, but might choose not to because they seem not to be worth living? When it is clear that death would be a welcome outcome to a tragic case, what are the limits of what we may do to facilitate it? Is it fair to make patients contribute to the costs of medical education and research through the mechanisms of billing for health care services? If not, how can they be adequately supported? And so on.

These considerations provide little comfort concerning the conflict over abortion policy. Instead of moving us closer to a stable resolution of that conflict, they seem only to illuminate the insuperable barriers to resolution. But perhaps there can be at least an indirect benefit; perhaps understanding why resolution is elusive can diminish the fervor with which the various partisans advocate their positions. I can't be very optimistic about that; people who are convinced that they know the right way are notoriously hard to defuse. But we would all be better off, as Smith suggests, if we could come to think of a contemplated abortion more as an occasion of personal crisis demanding a sensitive and caring response, and less as a matter of concern in the forums of public policy.

Such increased understanding of other peoples' motives, even if we are unable to accept their substantive positions, will be an important asset in a very difficult effort—the effort to deal with ongoing controversies about human reproduction in a way that preserves a tolerably harmonious social order.

.5.
FAILING ORGANS

The process of aging brings with it a gradual deterioration of physical functioning that in turn can have cognitive and psychological consequences. If all systems diminish in parallel, so that we age with perfectly uniform deterioration, we will be like the wonderful one-horse shay—functioning until everything wears out and falls apart at once. We will reach, in approaching that final moment, the seventh stage described so classically by Shakespeare in *As You Like It:* ". . . and mere oblivion, Sans teeth, sans eyes, sans taste, sans everything."

Such a harmonious demise is rare, since people more typically die of diseases or systemic defects that strike primarily at a specific physiological system. Such possible causes of death are many; perhaps a fatal neurological or hematological condition, perhaps a malignancy or immunological weakness, possibly a circulatory deficiency. Often, it is the failure of a single vital organ, such as a kidney, heart, or liver—each of which serves a specific and distinctive systemic function that is necesary for continued survival. Such organ failure can come at any age, striking people who are otherwise in sound physical condition.

Until very recently, the failure of any vital organ was invariably fatal. In our time, it has become possible to fix organs that are broken, to substitute machines that will serve their functions for them, and even to replace them with organs from elsewhere. This is high technology, high drama, "rescue" medicine. It is extremely costly, and raises a host of intriguing issues.

In addition to the transplantation of kidneys (sometimes with the pancreas as well), Boston's Beth Israel provides medical management of many patients who are at risk for organ failure. It also performs open heart surgery and it has a major renal dialysis unit. There is widespread interest within the hospital in all aspects of health care's capacity to respond to the failure of vital organs.

The issues surrounding the use of dialysis machines are particularly instructive. This treatment has a special place in the history of modern bioethics, for kidney dialysis first brought to widespread public attention that new medical capacities bring new moral dilemmas.

A dialysis machine, or "artificial kidney," is essentially a washing machine for the blood. It is connected via tubes to the patient's circulatory system so that the blood detours out of the body, travels through the machine, and returns. The machine filters out the toxic wastes that are naturally produced by the body, which will kill the patient within a matter of days if they are not removed. In a healthy person, the kidney does that essential job; when it fails, the machine can do the job instead. What requires technical wizardry is getting the filtration just right—removing the waste while allowing the valuable contents of the blood to escape filtration. The process is slow and its benefits are brief. So a patient on dialysis must be connected to the machine for several hours at a time, several days a week. The relationship between patient and machine is not just technically sophisticated, but psychologically complex, at once saving the patient's life and converting it to a life of unremitting dependency.

In 1964, in a widely read article in *Life Magazine*, Shana Alexander described the problem of selecting those patients who would be given access to the few places available in Seattle's pioneering renal dialysis unit. She thus underscored the need to make decisions about how the life-saving capacities of modern medicine should be allocated.

The thought of turning patients away to die who could be saved with a machine that has been developed, but is just not widely available, prompts an almost automatic reply: make more of those machines. That is, of course, just what happened. In addition to great technical improvement in dialysis equipment over the last two and a half decades, the machines have been made widely available, so that no medically qualified patient must die for lack of available equipment. Even the cost is no barrier, since the federal government's End Stage Renal Disease program covers the costs of the treatment of kidney failure. So the problems of rationing show up elsewhere now—for example, in the debate about the costs of the artificial heart or in the task of selecting transplant recipients for scarce organs or organ combinations—and not in the dialysis unit, where a more likely source of distress is the suspicion that too many people are on dialysis.

The staff of the dialysis unit assembles around coffee and doughnuts in a very small conference room. I am just here to observe, to listen to what they talk about at these meetings. But my presence again distorts the conversation; as soon as they hear from the unit director what my agenda is, they change theirs.

Most of them are highly trained nurses who specialize in dialysis. Their hours are good; there is no night shift on the unit. But they have their frustrations. "The hardest thing," one of them emphasizes, "is to treat someone repetitively with zero *gain." Although the dialysis patients here are on average eleven years older than the average for dialysis patients generally, she is most frustrated by a teen-ager on the unit.*

He has AIDS, and is failing fast. Earlier, he was hostile and combative, and the nurses approached him with caution and anxiety—not so much because of the AIDS, but because of his aggressiveness. But now he is almost comatose, with just inter-mittent periods of marginal lucidity. A second nurse also hates to care for him; she knows that he is dying, and wonders what the point can be of prolonging his decline. "Are we doing anything for him or just to him?" she asks, echoing once again the pervasive dilemma of highly sophisticated health care.

I ask about his family; they are keeping vigil. "But families rarely come to the dialysis unit," a nurse informs me. "Many families don't ever see it." I had no idea; I had assumed that the families of patients on dialysis would be well informed about dialysis and would become involved themselves in helping the patients endure their sessions on the machine. At the very least, I thought, they would want to see what happened in the strange environment to which the patient was so inextricably tied for so many hours a week. I am startled to discover this evidence of families distancing themselves from the patients' experience, avoiding the discomfort of confronting the patient's discomfort, dependency, and, perhaps, deterioration or despair. What, I wonder, is it really like out there, outside the conference room, where the patients are?

But I must wait a little longer to find out; the staff members are eager to explain more to me about the stresses they must bear in the face of difficult decisions. One man, I learn, said "No more dialysis" and was dead in three days. He'd had enough, made his choice, and his choice was honored. None of the unit staff have any misgivings about that case. But, they explain, legal complexities can inhibit withdrawal of dialysis. They tell of a man with no next of kin who was doing well on dialysis, but then had a massive stroke. He had often orally expressed his preferences not to be sustained under such conditions, but there was no written record of those expressions. The medical director of the unit went to court to have a guardian ad litem appointed. Six weeks later, after conducting a panel review of the case, the guardian found that dialysis should be continued. "He didn't want it, and we didn't want to be doing it to him. But we had to keep doing it," a nurse laments. Once again, I am reminded that it is important not just to express one's preferences, but to establish a written record of them.

"And often the family puts a lot of pressure on a patient to continue," she adds. "They don't spend time here seeing what it's like, but they insist that nobody give up."

"Yes," explains the medical director, "that's true. And sometimes it is because of guilt, but sometimes it is real devotion."

At last we move into the unit. But not because our discussion has ended. It is only that time is running short, and we must move on. I have said very little; just my being present as "the ethics guy" has apparently allowed the staff to pour out their frustrations more extensively than they typically have time for. My being there has legitimized an agenda they are very eager to pursue.

On the unit, I am struck by the unexpected diversity of the patients. Jim is a middle-aged employee of a local television *station. His hours are flexible, so he can work full-time and still arrange for his dialysis sessions. He is doing extremely well, and is ambivalent about the idea of a transplant. They have benefits, but also problems, and his present situation is stable and entirely tolerable.*

Sadie just screams. "Totally out of it," says one of the nurses. There's no reason to think she is in pain, and it doesn't matter what they do to or for her. Sadie screams.

Jeri is stable on dialysis; betweeen treatments she goes home and takes drugs. She's an addict.

Dan is in his early thirties. He had a transplant, quickly rejected; a second transplant worked well for nine years and then failed. How silly of me to have assumed that if they worked well for a year or two, they'd be good for the duration. Dan is waiting for a third transplant, even though he developed a seizure disorder as a by-product of the previous one. He is in good spirits, is fully employed, but does not want to remain dependent on the machine.

Old Mr. Nolan is of uncertain antiquity. He has only one leg and no teeth. His eyes sparkle with good cheer, an immense toothless grin dominates his grizzled face, and he shakes with laughter at the TV screen before him.

Max stares glumly, blankly. The doctor tells me that Max has repeatedly said "No more dialysis." But his family pressures him to keep coming in. "What is our responsibility here?" asks the doctor. "Should we support the patient's position? Do we stay out of it? Do we side with the family? These are very hard questions for us to face."

Because there is no shortage of money or machines for the treatment of kidney patients, dialysis has become a standard therapy. In the mid-1960s it was unusual for a patient with kidney failure to be placed on dialysis; now the prevailing expectation favors dialysis, and withholding or withdrawing it requires serious justification. It is no longer a scarce resource, and some have even argued that its ready availability without cost to patients, and in some settings with substantial potential profit to providers, has led to extensive overuse of the therapy.

Dialysis provides another example of the development of a positive good, much sought after while scarce, which may have become transformed through its greater availability into a treatment that is now imposed on some patients in an almost conventional way, sometimes with insufficient grounding in the particular needs, values, and interests of the individual patient. Now that we have learned how to provide dialysis to everyone who needs it, we also need the capacity to recognize that even though it once was scarce, it isn't necessarily always a benefit now.

The new treatment of choice, transplantation, has replaced dialysis as a focus of concern about scarcity. It is one thing to say "make more machines," quite another to say "get more transplantable organs." Much has been written about the problems of allocating the transplantable organs that are available and about increasing the supply. The more extreme proposals have included a plan—now, fortunately, prohibited by law—that there be a commercial market within which poor people could make money by selling one of their kidneys. And some have proposed that tax incentives be provided to those who allow their organs to be made available, or even that suitable organs be usable for transplantation unless the deceased had expressly dissented while alive. But the prevailing sentiment, at least for the time being, favors increased public education as the mechanism most apporpriate for increasing the supply of transplantable organs of all kinds.

The eagerness of hospitals to obtain organs for transplantation from donors increases with the technical ability to use such organs successfully. That eagerness is echoed in public policy; in New York State it is required by law that hospital personnel ask the next of kin for permission to use the transplantable organs of those who die under their jurisdiction. The capacity to transplant organs singly and in combinations, in addition to skin, muscle, bone, and corneas, despite its remarkable development in recent years, may be just a beginning. We may yet see the day when whole limbs and other complex physiological systems are considered replaceable parts. But the costs of the development of these capacities are unfathomable.

Even the development of mechanical substitutes for vital organs does not solve the problem of scarcity of resources. The ready availability of dialysis machines has drawn the fatal sting from end stage renal failure, but, in part because of the problems of imposed or subtly coercive use of the treatment, the cost has been far more than the government anticipated in undertaking to finance the treatment.

Such economic considerations may underlie the fact that, having committed to the support of treatment for kidney failure, the federal government has declined to provide similar protection to patients of any other kind. Heart failure, like kidney failure, can strike anyone. Why should the cost of its treatment not be similarly covered by a federal program? The answer must surely lie in the judgment that, despite the good that such a program would do for individual patients, the collective effect of bearing the immense costs would, on balance, be socially and politically undesirable. And the costs would be immense, because there are a great many people with treatable heart conditions who would have been untreatable just a few decades ago.

By the time I arrive at the surgical unit, the patient is already in the operating room, prepared for surgery. In my gown and mask, I look like the rest of the crowd. But there is a major difference; I have never been in an OR before, and I am very uncertain about how well this is going to go. Blood and guts were no particular strong point of mine; I survived my one high school biology course, but never entertained as much as a single premedical thought.

My host, Dr. L, is one of the anesthesiologists. We agreed to meet today at 7:30, but it wasn't clear which patient we would see, or what sort of surgery. That vagueness helps sustain my commitment to do this, along with the belief that it is something I ought to do and the fear of being utterly embarrassed by backing out. But any enthusiasm I appear to have is pure theater. Dr. L is reassuring; he tells me not to worry, and says that any reaction I can have would be familiar to the staff and easily handled. (I interpret this as proof that observers regularly get sick, faint away, or otherwise make nuisances of themselves. I feel doomed.)

"Okay. So what are we going to see today?" I inquire as we head from the locker room toward the operating room.

"It's a cabbage and valve," he replies. I understand the lingo: a cabbage is a CABG—a coronary arterial bypass graft. So the valve is a heart valve. We are heading toward open heart surgery. I had

hoped to start with, maybe, a bunion. I glance about, checking escape routes as we enter the OR.

The patient is a man of 81. Heavily sedated, he nods a groggy greeting to me from the table, as the crowd in the room grows larger. Dr. L introduces me to various members of the support staff—the anesthesiologist who will be working on the case, nurses, surgical residents, technicians. There is an air of bustling about, of preparation, that reminds me of backstage just before curtain time. The star, I suppose, is the heart surgeon who will appear later, in the second act, after the patient has already undergone the first stages of the surgery.

Now, these first stages are underway. The patient's bodily functions are under the control of the anesthesiologist, who stands near the patient's head at a large console of instruments, valves, switches, and lights. I forget about being backstage, and think of the pilot bringing in a 747 in bad weather.

The younger surgeons have cut a long incision in the patient's right leg; they will remove a length of vein to be used to create the new vessels to the heart. Soon, another surgeon will open the chest cavity, cutting along a thin line drawn on a plastic film that now covers the patient's chest. Dr. L warns me that a small electric saw is used to cut through the sternum. Before I can react, he takes me by the arm and guides me toward the head of the table. A small vertical screen separates the torso from the neck and head, so the scene of action seems oddly detached from any actual person. I peer over the shoulder of one of the doctors, squinting self-protectively. But I can see very well.

Dr. L slides a short stepping-stool past the control console right to the head of the table. "Stand up here; you can see better," he says, leading me up onto the stool. I am perhaps three feet from the site of the incision as the whining saw blade starts to cut through the sternum. I think, "You have just two choices. You stand here, and watch carefully and see how this is done. Or you fall over. If you fall over, there are two ways you can fall. You can fall into the control panel, wrecking it and killing the patient, in which case many people are furious and it is a great embarrassment. Or you can fall the other way, landing in the incision, killing the patient directly, which is also nothing to be proud of." Before I can decide, the chest cavity is open, and I am staring, awed, at a beating human heart.

Soon the principal surgeon is at work. The patient's circulatory and respiratory functions have been transferred via connecting tubes to a dual-speaker AM-FM stereo cassette heart-lung machine, which has been the source of the OR's music all along. The operator of the machine controls such things—in addition to the music—as the rate of flow of the patient's blood, its temperature, and its oxygen level. By cooling the blood, it is possible to place the patient in what is almost a state of suspended animation, lowering greatly the risk of brain damage due to oxygen deprivation and otherwise minimizing the impact of the disconnection of the natural heart.

To control the bleeding at various points, the doctors cauterize the ends of small blood vessels with an electric device. I am unprepared for the smell, the acrid consequence of cooking small bits of the patient to a crisp. The absence of this smell from films and videotapes of surgery makes them utterly lack a powerful part of the reality of the event. Fortunately, the barbecue is brief.

The surgeon is examining the vein from the patient's leg, selecting pieces for the replacement graft. All four vessels will be done, so four lengths are needed. Why, I wonder, is he painting a thin blue stripe down the side of each piece?

The surgeons peer intently into the chest cavity, discussing how best to proceed. They know the results of various imaging procedures, but those results are always somewhat impressionistic. There is apparently no substitute for opening up the patient and seeing the details of what it is really like in there. What it is really like in there today is a bit different, a bit tighter, than what was expected. The surgeons are a bit surprised by how this patient's innards are laid out. They discuss and agree on their approach, and proceed to the grafting. They take care to see that each stripe is straight, ensuring that the length of vein is not twisted and subject to unwanted torsion. That done, they must replace the faulty valve. The new one will be a porcine valve—a valve from the heart of a pig, used to repair the heart of a man! And the man is active in a local synagogue. I chuckle to myself at the thought of a kosher life saved by a piece of pork!

With consummate delicacy, the principal surgeon opens the heart and cuts out the old valve. When the site is prepared, he asks for the new valve. It comes in a small blue jar, and the cover is on very tightly. A nurse tries to open the jar, then hands it to the nearest assemblage of surgical gown and mask that appears to contain a male. Inside that assemblage I wonder, as I loosen the cover, "Am I allowed to participate *in this?*

The surgery, which lasted seven hours, was entirely successful. Over the next ten days, I visited the patient almost daily; I felt that I had an investment in his recovery and wanted to learn more about his motivation and aspirations. He did well, and was up and about in a few days. But his recovery was not as fast as that of many younger patients; it was nearly two weeks before he went home. Sometimes we sat and swapped jokes; he'd heard them all. Sometimes he talked about his family or his business and his eagerness to return to work. He was vital, forward looking, and in very good spirits most of the time. The only discouragement I saw resulted from impatience on his part to regain his strength, and that was due to unrealistic hopes that soon passed. I enjoyed the luxury of having time to spend with "my patient," and was pleased not to be one of the doctors who, having performed their surgical wizardry, moved promptly on to other patients without much chance to savor the results of their work.

But why should they be as impressed as I? Such operations are now routine. It is major surgery, to be sure, but of a sort that is performed tens of thousands of times a year, with a very high rate of success. And it is a mild measure indeed, compared with heart transplantation. Yet even that has become an accepted medical practice in carefully circumscribed situations, and has recently been included within the coverage of some medical insurance plans. At the same time, artificial hearts, despite the vast problems associated with them, are an experimental reality.

In considering the further development of an artificial heart, it is important to distinguish the question of whether an artificial heart is beneficial therapy for a particular patient from the very different question of whether an artificial heart program is a wise choice for societal support. The answer is unclear at both levels.

That program is costly and highly complex, its progress has

been uneven at best, and it has been controversial—with its most ardent supporters holding that it merits continued public funding, while its most severe critics argue that it is an extravagant example of medical technophilia run wild. The debate involves difficult questions of social policy.

A series of choices by individuals in a community, each of which is to the advantage of those individuals—for example, the farmer, the manufacturer, or the patient—may have collective effects that are to the disadvantage of the entire community. And a program that benefits each recipient may not benefit the social order.

Was Barney Clark, the first recipient of an artificial heart, well served by the treatment he received? That continues to be a matter of dispute. (Some of his physicians have referred to him consistently as their "co-investigator," rather than as their patient.) Even if he or other recipients of the device did clearly benefit, does the program constitute a wise social choice?

Roger Evans, writing about the economic constraints on high technology medical care, offers gloomy predictions.* He distinguishes between resource allocation and resource rationing—the first is the determination of a level of support for a program; the second is the determination of which subset of those in need will receive benefits provided by the program. He then argues that "It is now apparent that both resource allocation and resource rationing decisions will become inevitable. . . . The demand for health care will doubtlessly outstrip available resources. . . . Persons will be recognized as in need of, and then denied, benefits that the medical care system is capable of providing."

Such predictions, and the reasons for them, cast a pall of concern over the health care providers at Boston's Beth Israel, and throughout the health care professions, because of the threat they pose to the long cherished goal of making medical need the sole determinant of access to medical care. Evans' unpleasant conclusions are followed by a discussion of criteria for allocation and rationing, including the suggestion that the availability of health care be based in part not on medical need but on some measure of

* Roger W. Evans, "Health Care Technology and the Inevitability of Resource Allocation and Rationing Decisions, I, II," *Journal of the American Medical Association,* April 15, 1983, 249 (15), 2047–53; and April 22/29, 1983 (16), 2208–19.

worthiness. Evans writes, "Ultimately . . . the limits of the broad humanistic concept of a right to health care must be recognized. Within the context of rationing, those persons who have done the most to preserve their health could conceivably be the first to benefit from the available resources." After all, one might argue, there is a link of shared responsibility between patients and the social context that makes medical care available, in respect both to its development and covering its costs.

With these discomforting observations as background, consider a few aspects of the program to develop an artificial heart. Pierre Galletti argues that "fear of an imminent major impact on health care services and costs is not justified (*New England Journal of Medicine*, February 1, 1984). Yet the *New York Times* (January 15, 1983), in an editorial about totally implantable devices, worries that a successful artificial heart program would cost $3 billion per year (assuming 34,000 recipients annually), and conjectures that "There may well be more sensible ways to spend that kind of money." Barton Bernstein projects the cost as being in the range of $1.6 to $6.6 billion per year, and calls for "a probing public dialogue about the costs—economic and social—of developing this device (*The Nation*, January 22, 1983). So there is substantial dispute about just what is at stake economically. But there are other issues as well.

Whether an artificial heart benefits a particular patient is not solely a medical question. Physicians can assess the extent to which the treatment fulfills their aspirations, but the patient's independent assessment is crucial, as Dr. Robert Jarvik has pointed out in discussing Dr. Clark's case. This is so precisely because the aspirations of patient and physician can easily diverge in a case of this sort, and a due regard for the patient requires us to guard against mistaking physicians' goals for those of the patient.

Assuming that there is genuine benefit to individual patients, whether the overall program is societally worth pursuing is a new and thoroughly nonmedical question. Medical judgments are not irrelevant; but neither are they decisive. They are merely important data in the context of a social policy debate. We cannot conclude that it is good to have any particular program on the grounds that each instance of treatment under that program can be reasonably expected to be good, considered separately. We need to make such judgments on the basis of collective concerns. But that is something we do not yet know very well how to do.

Even if a program of artificial heart treatment is generally worth pursuing, serious problems remain. For example, as philosopher Gerald Dworkin has noted, by making something possible, we sometimes unwittingly make it necessary or, at least, difficult to avoid even where it is not likely to be a benefit.* We may to some extent have done that already in the case of dialysis. The availability of an artificial heart would generate a coercive pressure on patients to pursue that remedy and on families to provide it. Neither might be able to muster the temerity, in the face of a vital crisis, to challenge the assumption that what can be done should be done. Yet one can easily imagine an unexpressed preference all around for spurning such heroic efforts. This is not a conclusive objection to the development of any new capacity, but it is an often inadequately recognized consequence of progress.

So failing organ systems no longer need be fatal. The array of remedies is rapidly growing. In the case of Baby Fae, which led to vigorous public debate, we have even seen the effort to save a child's life by means of a xenograft—the transplanting of a baboon's heart into a human infant. Where will it all end? Where should it end?

The short-lived Baby Fae made an even bigger splash with her transplanted baboon's heart than the USDA's notorious experiments inserting human genes into sheep and pigs to make them grow larger. We have used heart valves from pigs to repair human hearts for years—more than 100,000 times—without anybody getting excited about species mixing. But baboon hearts! This time, have we gone too far? For that matter, have we gone too far with high technology medicine generally, or with genetic engineering outside the medical realm?

How should we think about such questions? Consider as examples of that general problem the two hypothetical reports below. Should we applaud them? Are they a fate we should dread? Or are they perhaps a fantasy we should dismiss as having no realistic bearing on the choices actually before us?

* Gerald Dworkin, "Is More Choice Better Than Less?" *Midwest Studies in Philosophy, v. 7, Social and Political Philosophy, ed.* P. French, T. Uehling, Jr., and H. Wettstein (Minneapolis: University of Minnesota Press, 1982).

1. *Avant-garde Hospital today reported a major breakthrough in the treatment of accident victims. Four-year-old Girl Grace, riding her tricycle along the sidewalk, lost her balance and fell into the path of a truck that drove over her right arm, destroying it. Grace was rushed to the shock-trauma unit, where a surgical team, noted for its pioneering successes in reattaching the severed limbs of accident victims, grafted the arm of a young baboon onto her body. Now, improved immunosuppressant drugs and promising animal experiments have led to optimism that Grace, and others like her, will have functional digits and limbs despite the severity of their accidents.*

A hospital spokesman said, "We anticipate that, if the grafting is successful, Girl Grace will require some special counseling as she is growing up. But she will have two functioning arms! This new therapy does not save lives like the transplantation of vital organs. But it brings the patient closer to normal functioning, which is what most medical treatment is about. So we're very excited about it."

2. *The Defense Department revealed today that genetic engineers, working on a top secret enterprise on the scale of the Manhattan Project, have bred a new class of footsoldier. The Pentagon's statement said, in part, "These new warriors greatly enhance our ability to secure peace through strength. They have immense stamina, physical strength, and resistance to pain. Within the range of their abilities, they follow instructions superbly. They mature quickly and have marvelous, uncomplaining dispositions.*

The scientific foundation that makes this great advance possible was the complete mapping of the human genome in the mid-1990s. The nation is indebted to the dedicated scientists who, over the intervening thirty years, have worked with genetic material from great athletes, mentally handicapped people, primates, and certain other mammals, learning to combine that material into this crucial part of the greatest force for peace the world has ever known.

How much of this sort of development—the first involving transplants and the second gene-mixing—is defensible? How can we assess the ethics of these possibilities?

We should begin, at least, by reasoning carefully, respecting important distinctions, and withholding judgments that exceed the warrant of the facts. There's little point in simply shouting back and forth at one another; we need policy decisions that will serve us all well. For how the growing debate comes out will affect not only what medical cures will be available for failing organs and other medical problems, but even what kinds of beings there are and what humans will look like.

One complaint about Baby Fae's transplant contends that it was an abuse of the baboon. The moral character of our relationship to animals *is* important, and is receiving the increased attention and clarification it deserves. Nonetheless, for the sake of argument, accept the most prevalent sentiment on this point: Provided no other treatment is comparably promising, the baboon's interests are not alone sufficient for opposing such transplant surgery.

Other complaints said that the transplant was flawed technology—that it was not the best available treatment, was not sufficiently promising even in the absence of any other option, and was done without adequately informed parental consent. These are all reasonable objections, but they distract us from considering the propriety of interspecies transfer. So, again, assume that the treatment cannot be opposed on such grounds.

We are left with the fundamental objection that seemed to cause the emotional response—that such transplantation is wrong because it violates the integrity of natural species—wrong inherently just because it is species mixing. Advocates of such a view speak of "the rights of each species to exist as a separate, identifiable creature," and cite the respect for species integrity that is reflected in our endangered species laws.

In the aftermath of Baby Fae, however, we have learned how common it has become to use animal parts to repair humans, even their hearts. Why then was there so much fuss about Baby Fae?

Some of it surely arises from the symbolic significance of the heart. On the one hand, the heart is just a vital organ—one of the simpler ones, at that. It is primarily a pump, little more. If it fails, the challenge is to fix or replace it. That task is prominent on the agenda of medical science and in the public consciousness because lots of hearts fail.

Ah, but then there is the other hand. For lots of hearts break, as well. And what would romantic poetry be without the heart? Could Lovelace have conveyed the impact of Gratiana's dancing by writing, "And when she ceas'd, we sighing saw the floor lay pav'd with broken spleens?"

Would you want a valentine that said "I love you with all my liver?"

Would you rush to see a film named *Kind Kidneys and Coronets?*

Our language and mythology imbue the heart with metaphorical power that shapes our emotional reactions to medical news. But cool reflection should lead us to separate the one hand from the other, and to make judgments about medical care strictly on the basis of relevant considerations.

So we reject the notion that all species mixing therapies are inherently wrong, recognizing that we have relied on them comfortably already. And we reject the charge that Baby Fae's transplant was wrong just because it was a heart, rather than some other organ, or just because it was a whole heart, rather than only a valve.

Are we then left unable to object to any future interspecies transplant that seems to be the best available option from the perspective of medical technology? Are we committed to accepting the xenographic treatment of Girl Grace?

I think not. But if we are to resist it, we ought to be able to distinguish it from the cases we accept. We ought to be able to say something credible about why it is different.

Forget that it is not technically feasible today to graft a primate's limb onto a person. That could change quickly in any case. Assume no robotic limb could achieve comparable functional capacity. If the patient were your daughter, would you grant consent for the primate graft? I would not, and I was fairly sure of that before I had any clear idea why not.

British philosopher Jonathan Glover, in his book *What Sort of People Should There Be?*, helps shed some light on the matter. "Our present practice is to act in quite different ways towards humans and towards members of other species," he writes. If we were to blur "the clear gap between monkeys and ourselves," we would face the need to develop appropriate patterns of behavior toward the resulting beings. And they would have to find ways of relating to us. It could be very difficult.

Baby Fae, had she lived, would have been unmistakably human, despite her heart. (Her elementary school chums, knowing her history, would have denied it, but that is a separate matter.) Girl Grace, however, would be unmistakably anomalous. She would live surrounded by people who struggled to know what to make of her, how to react to her. She would live behind a wall of strangeness, making normal relationships impossible: Would you (or would you expect your brother or son to) date a girl with a baboon arm?

Of course, we do establish relationships, often less naturally and comfortably than we should, with those who visibly fall far outside the range of normal human body images because of injury, illness, or congenital anomaly. We know that their character and worth transcend the limitations of their bodies, and we know it is our own limitations that introduce awkwardness into our dealings with them.

Yet we also know that participation in the human social order is deeply rooted in having a human body. A body visibly constructed from the parts of other animals is one that we would respond to in a fundamentally different way than to a body that nature has misshapen, or that man has supplemented with machine-like prosthetics. So the thought of doctors *creating* such a body *on purpose* causes us to be revulsed or made very anxious. We know better how to deal with amputees than with Girl Grace; they know better how to deal with us.

I have no *proof* that Girl Grace's operation is a bad idea. It is a matter of judgment, supported by reasons which can be persuasive without being conclusive. But even if you are not persuaded in this particular case—even if you could gracefully accept your child having a baboon arm, surely you can imagine some combination of animal parts attached to a human brain that you would be unable to accept as totally human. Then somewhere along the continuum from the unproblematic pig valve to that unacceptable combination, the balance has shifted from "yes" to "no."

One objection may be that this position seems to sanction an assessment of human worth based on externals—that it defines a person's humanity in terms of visible appearance rather than character, rationality, and psychological capacity. After all, many severely deformed people not only function in society, but humble, instruct, and inspire us with their courage, tenacity, and accomplishment.

But the objection is a misunderstanding. I do not propose to diminish our respect for the *victims* of severe deformation due to accidents of birth or circumstance. I simply propose to acknowledge that they *are* victims, and to resist similarly victimizing others knowingly, when we have a choice, by increasing their separation from their fellow human beings, thus diminishing their humanity.

Critics challenge this sort of position by asking, "Where do we draw the line between 'yes' and 'no'?" They point to another recent issue in current medicine—gene therapy—fearing that if we start altering genes to remove a congenital defect, we will become committed to a brutalizing quest for genetically engineered human perfection.

The new breed of hybrid warrior would be clearly forbidden by the criterion I have suggested; we could not relate to such a consciously designed product as totally human. Yet I welcome the gene therapy presently under development.

No one now at work in genetic engineering intends to develop medical interventions that will modify the complex heritable character—the germline—of humans. Nor can anyone think of any practical way to develop such a technology that would reliably produce beneficial results.

The gene therapy now planned is a way to help patients who suffer from specific, genetically based, deadly diseases such as Lesch-Nyan disease—the victims of which uncontrollably shred their own flesh as they deteriorate. This kind of therapy is called "somatic"—it treats an individual suffering from genetic disease without in any way affecting his or her offspring. In this way, the technology is not ethically different from plastic surgery to "cure" a person of having a disagreeable facial characteristic, without affecting that person's offspring's likelihood of having such a feature.

No proposals for human germline intervention, as opposed to somatic therapy, are under development. The medical researchers at the forefront of genetic therapy have affirmed their aversion to any use of genetic techniques for germline intervention or for enhancement of normal functioning, as contrasted with the repair of serious genetic defects associated with life-threatening or debilitating disease.

It is foolish—indeed, cruel—to oppose the responsible development of beneficial somatic therapies on the ground that projects of a sort not now underway could lead to bad outcomes if we were unable, once they were underway, to set sensible policies of limitation. It would also be foolish to assume that no surveillance is needed of developments in genetic engineering, interspecies transfer, or other exotic remedies for failing organs. What is learned by advances in somatic therapy, for example, *could* lead to progress toward germline intervention, and that *could* lead to socially and ethically unpalatable consequences. But we need not fear that outcome, so long as we separate fact from fantasy, and openly debate the limits that should constrain our emerging skills.

Those who argue differently are devotees of the "slippery slope" approach. The structure of their argument is familiar: What is now contemplated may seem justifiable by itself, but it is the first step toward an intolerable outcome. If we allow that first step, we will have no way to halt the process, for drawing any line of limitation will be arbitrary and controversial. So we must not allow the first step. Such "slippery slope" arguments are sometimes sound, but often they are not. Each instance must be assessed on its merits.

Consider: if we allow research on human subjects, people will be exploited and harmed in the interest of medical progress. Yet we have drawn the line; we have an elaborate, imperfect, but largely successful set of guidelines and mechanisms to protect the subjects of medical research. The kinds of abuses of human research subjects that occurred in the past have essentially now been eliminated.

Consider: if we allow abortion without limit in the first trimester, we will lose all respect for life and will accept infanticide of any unwanted infant. That argument has been heard, but despite a liberal abortion policy, we have not moved even slightly in the direction of indifference toward infanticide. Indeed, our efforts to protect children from abuse and deprivation of all kinds seem to be more vigorous than ever.

The slippery slope arguments against interspecies transplants and gene transfer are not very good. It is easy to envision a distasteful outcome from unrestrained applications of any technical advance. But there is no need for the gloomy view that restraint is impossible. Our record is better than that.

Assume that curing an individual's genetic disease is, in principle, justifiable, and that the creation of hybrid soldiers is not. How can we defend a policy that says "yes" to the former and "no" to the latter? Where do we draw the line, and why?

No man turns from hirsute to bald when one last, crucial hair departs. There's a region between the clear cases in which it is impossible, and also unnecessary, to decide whether baldness has been achieved. Similarly, a man with a pig's valve in his heart is entirely human (you still have the same car even if you replace the alternator), but a human head transplanted onto the body of an ape would clearly be an interspecies hybrid (you would not have the same car if you kept only the engine and replaced everything else). Between, there are regions of grey, where it is impossible to make the call.

Arguments based on the question "Where do you draw the line?" try to capitalize on that impossibility. The crucial point that they miss is that *it doesn't matter* where exactly such lines are drawn, so long as they include the clearly tolerable cases and rule out the clearly intolerable ones. Draw them anywhere, after suitable public debate, so long as they fall within the band of grey that separates black from white cases. Once we recognize that it is unnecessary to draw the line precisely, we need no longer be distressed that it is impossible to do so. There is a range within which judgment must be made, and that we can often do.

We've done that with abortion policy—a good example precisely because there is such bitter dispute about it. The overwhelming majority position is that newborn infants count as people and that the day-old embryo does not. Somewhere between, personhood emerges gradually, as the fetus develops the neurological capacity for cognition and sentience.

Personhood does not just snap into place, so we cannot cite a special point at which it is suddenly present. By allowing abortions

early in this process of development, but resisting them later, the
Supreme Court in *Roe* v. *Wade* (albeit on different reasoning) has
drawn a line appropriately through a murky band of grey that
separates two situations so different in degree as to be different in
kind, despite the continuity of process that leads from one to the
other.

I would oppose interspecies transplantation procedures that
produce what, on reflection, we cannot comfortably conclude is
clearly human in the interpersonally most significant respects.
Others would set the limits somewhat differently. I trust that after
open debate about the issues, public sentiment would favor a
policy close enough to that to satisfy me. More organs might be
transplanted between species, but disfiguring hybridization of
Grace's kind would be widely opposed. Some would complain that
the limits were too severe and hindered potentially beneficial
medical progress. Indeed, several commentators on the views I
have expressed here have criticized them as too restrictive. Others
would complain that the limits were too lax, and violated various
moral strictures. But most of us would be content that we had
found a way into the medical future that struck an acceptable
balance. That's how public policy should proceed in such matters—with a search on all sides for an accommodation within the
band of grey, although the effort is only sometimes successful.

To say all this is to place great reliance on our capacity to
exercise judgment. It is to respect our ability to face an uncertain
future, confident that we can bring reason to bear on new possibilities, to separate progress from madness. It is to say that we dare
proceed, because we can exercise discretion, change direction,
and say, when we have to, "This far is far enough. Here, we shall
stop." We need to do all that with regard to high technology health
care, genetic engineering, and a great many other social issues. I
have no proof that we will succeed. But we have the capacity, and
need only to develop the resolve to do so.

I have been raising some questions about the treatment of
failing organs. But a caution is needed here. There is a tradition of
valuing the raising of questions, even where we have no clear
sense of how to answer them. This, at least on some accounts, is a
typical and valuable part of the philosopher's stock-in-trade. It is
always good, we sometimes think, to anticipate questions we may

have to face in the future; the harder they will be to answer, the greater the value of raising them early.

But some questions are better unasked, and surely better unanswered. Here's an example: at one point, in the face of severe fiscal uncertainty, senior administrators at my former university felt the need to engage in contingency planning. That was reasonable enough. But then the word came down; department heads were to state explicitly what they would do in the event of budget cuts of various degrees of stringency. Answering the question as it was asked would have meant identification of those faculty members in the greatest peril of being dismissed. The only tolerable response to that administrative directive was a flat refusal to comply. To identify particular faculty members—even to oneself—as the ones who hypothetically would be selected as most dispensable would be actually to incur damage, of a potentially lasting sort, needlessly.

I recall that episode as I consider the prospect of rationing sophisticated treatment among medically qualified patients. Whom would we select in advance as the class of people we would be prepared if necessary to deny—people older than some specific maximum? Those who had engaged in clearly culpable behavior, such as smoking? What of the less clearly culpable, but still imprudent, heavy beef-eater, or the sedentary, or the workaholic? Or would we exclude those who fail a test of social utility or who are not wealthy enough to meet high costs?

These are familiar questions; some of them were faced in the early days of renal dialysis. They can also be destructive questions, for to answer them at all, even on the most tentative basis, is to devalue entire categories of people. We have set these questions aside in the case of renal dialysis, but only by adopting a very costly program of federal funding for all dialysis treatment. It seems highly unlikely that the same strategy can work for all other exotic treatments. We may, therefore, be unable in the end, as Roger Evans fears, to avoid such questions. But until we are unable to avoid them, it may be best to keep on trying.

A year after his heart surgery, the octogenarian patient whose operation I witnessed returned to see his internist. Their conversation, which was recorded, included this exchange:

Doctor: Have you been able to return to employment?

Patient: They can't keep me away. I go in nine-thirty; I stay maybe until four.

Doctor: So you work a full day?

Patient: No, I don't. I leave at four or four-thirty. Sometimes I stay until five or five-thirty, but that's my own fault.

Doctor: So you feel better than before your operation?

Patient: I feel a hundred percent better.

This patient's failing heart was repaired, and he has returned to an active, productive life at an age that until recently was considered quite advanced. In all likelihood, he will become a patient again, for one problem or another. If modern health care can continue to resolve his isolated medical problems as they arise, he will become more and more like that wonderful one-horse shay, wearing out slowly and broadly, rather than suddenly and sharply. Perhaps one day he will join the rapidly growing ranks of those who are very ill and very old, despite the earlier threat of a failing organ.

.6.
...

VERY ILL
AND
VERY OLD

I n 1985, the percentage of the population over 65 was 11%; in fewer than fifty years, that figure will approach 20%. The number of people over 85 will triple! According to a report issued by the National Institute on Aging, the number of Americans at least one hundred years old was approximately 25,000 in 1986, and will grow to 100,000 by the turn of the century! A generation hence, retirees will look forward as a matter of course to many decades of life, and people between 80 and 100 will be a much more significant segment of the population. Some of our centenarians are even still active and self-supporting. But health care is a problem for many of the very old already, and the magnitude of such problems will increase rapidly over the next several decades.

These problems are receiving increased attention in the public media, on a daily basis. The concerns of the very ill and very old are well illustrated, for example, by the articles in *The New York Times* of July 19, 1989. A front-page story reports that the suicide rate among elderly Americans increased by 25% from 1981 to 1986, even though "the elderly are generally more financially secure and healthier, and they live longer than their forbears." Many analysts attribute the trend to technological advances that extend life, but at a level of quality that is intolerable. The headline reads, "When Long Life Is Too Much: Suicide Rises Among the Elderly."

A second article (p. A14) concerns the Congressional debate about the surtax paid by many elderly Americans for insurance against the high costs of long-term hospitalization. And a third recounts the legal battle of Estelle M. Browning, who died at 89 "the way she never wanted to: in a nursing home, attached to a feeding tube." At issue is the deeply contested question of whether a written statement of objection to being kept alive by artificial means in the event of imminent death provides a justification for withdrawal of feeding tubes.

Boston's Beth Israel Hospital has many elderly patients. Some recover well enough that they no longer need hospital care, but not well enough that they can return to independent living. They must often be transferred to a long-term facility, typically a nursing home. Other patients have already been placed in nursing homes, from which they are admitted to the hospital in times of medical need that goes beyond what can be provided in the nursing homes. So there is a steady flow of patients between the hospital and the nursing homes, in both directions. Sometimes, patients' records are incomplete as a result of diverse admissions at different places; fragmented care and confusion about medication history can result.

I cross the bridge into Chelsea, glad to be heading outbound against the morning traffic, looking for the exit that will lead me to the Chelsea Jewish Nursing Home. I've been invited to spend the morning there, seeing a population that is not acutely ill, but with medical or functional problems making long-term care appropriate.

The building is modern and pleasant, renovated and expanded a few years ago after a very successful private funding campaign. My host, Dr. K, explains, as we head toward the first unit, that there are 120 residents, each of whom presents a set of problems somewhat different from those I see at the hospital. He introduces me to D, the nurse-practitioner with whom he works, and I listen as they discuss some of the patients.

The first issue to arise concerns Mr. H, who is not fully competent. He is in a hospital; his wife is here. As his next of kin, she has been asked to make a decision about some surgery that he should perhaps have. But she has had a stroke, is aphasic, and is not communicating well. So before the medical issues can be addressed directly, there are legal and bureaucratic entanglements to confront. It isn't enough for the medical staff at either the hospital or the nursing home to be clear about what ought to be done; they must see to it that the decision is made by someone who has definitive standing with respect to the patient—and that may take some doing. Without resolving the matter, we set out on rounds, starting in the room of a frail, elderly woman. Dr. K says, "Good morning, Mrs. Weston."

"Thank you so much for remembering my name," she replies. There is a bit of conversation about how she is doing, a brief examination, and then we leave.

In the hall, I ask D how old the patient is. The reply is more instructive than I had expected. "I don't know. Early eighties, maybe. I tend not to be very aware of their ages; I'm more concerned with their condition, their functional capacities, and their prospects."

Next, we see Mr. S, who, Dr. K tells me, is 102. He's had a rough go the last couple of years, and there has been on-going discussion about how aggressively he should be treated. He continues to relate to people to some extent, but has also been hospitalized on an emergency basis from time to time. One of his daughters favored a Do Not Resuscitate (DNR) order for him the last time, but the other daughter disagreed. Dr. K tells me, "I could have talked her into it, but she was really ambivalent, so I didn't."

As we walk on to the next floor, I ask D what her training has been; she tells me that it includes a number of years working in rehabilitation. She explains that a background in rehabilitation is invaluable in the nursing home setting. "A lot of standard rehabilitation stuff is not even thought of in most nursing homes," she laments. Her mission is not just to sustain these people, but to help them increase their functional capacities, even in the context of long-term care. I wonder at her dedication, sensitivity, and enthusiasm, and I wonder how many others like her there are. I suspect that she is a rare gem, and that to make her the norm would require greatly increased expenditure on nursing home care.

I look around as we walk along the corridor; two women sit in wheel chairs, staring blankly into the distance. They seem to have no interests or focus of attention. An elderly man, also in a wheel chair, looks straight ahead, repeating, "Doctor, Doctor, Doctor, Doctor. . . ."

I am struck by the immensity of the problem: the more we invest in the quality of these people's lives, the longer and better their lives can be, and the more it will cost to meet their needs and interests. If we become really effective at using the knowledge of rehabilitation specialists to improve the functioning of these frail, elderly people, they will probably live longer at a higher level of involvement. And that will increase the cost of sustaining them. So the better long-term care becomes, the worse the financial problem will become.

The recipients of long-term care include the chronically ill and seriously handicapped of all ages, but especially the aged. By most measures, that is the major category of need for long-term care, and that category is growing with alarming rapidity. In New York State, for example, there were 175,000 persons in residential long-term care facilities in 1988, with about 4000 more on the waiting lists.

And the situation is indeed alarming. As Robert Butler has said, we have barely begun to deal with the problems posed by an aging population. The sources of those problems include changing demographics, changing patterns of social organization, increased mobility of the population, a high divorce rate and the subsequent diffusion of social responsibility, the bureaucratization of social services, and even the successes of modern medicine.

What should the goals of long-term care be in facilities such as nursing homes? It is worth asking, because the answer makes a difference to what we do. Unless we know what aspirations are appropriate, it is impossible to evaluate our programs or our progress, or to know what changes to advocate.

Is the point of long-term care for the elderly to keep them alive longer, to make them more comfortable, to enrich their lives, to minimize their dependence on others, to minimize our investment in their continuing lives, to spare younger and more active people the burdens and distractions of caring for them at home? Each of these goals has something to be said for it, but each is to some extent in conflict with the others. What we decide to do depends on how we evaluate these and perhaps other goals in respect to one another. Indeed, what we decide to invest in the lives of the elderly will depend in part on how we judge their capacity to lead lives that are valuable to them. And that capacity will depend in turn on what we decide to invest in enriching their lives.

One common way of putting the question is in terms of justice in intergenerational transfer—what do we owe to the very elderly, and why? But that way of casting the question, although useful in some respects, also has the disadvantage of setting the issue in the language of "we" and "them," giving the illusion of a separation of constituencies that can distort the way we think about the matter. We, after all, given a bit of time and some good luck—will be them.

And what is it like to be them? The elderly have sometimes said the best claim that can be made for old age is that it is better than any known alternative. But it is not all of a piece; it is no more homogeneous that any other stage of life. And it is not necessarily all bad. Not all the very old are ill. Advanced age can be a time of sublime tranquility, beyond ambition and its attendant strains.

I had the good fortune many years ago to have Malcolm Cowley as my teacher, and I read his little volume *The View from 80* with great eagerness when it appeared. As usual, he puts the point particularly well:

> Those pleasures include some that younger people find hard to appreciate. One of them is simply sitting still, like a snake on a sun-warmed stone, with a delicious feeling of indolence that was seldom attained in earlier years. A leaf flutters down; a cloud moves by inches across the horizon. At such moments the older person, completely relaxed, has become a part of nature—and a living part, with blood coursing through his veins. The future does not exist for him. He thinks, if he thinks at all, that life for younger persons is still a battle royal of each against each, but that now he has nothing more to win or lose. He is not so much above as outside the battle, as if he had assumed the uniform of some small neutral country, perhaps Liechtenstein or Andorra. From a distance he notes that some of the combatants, men or women, are jostling ahead—but why do they fight so hard when the most they can hope for is a longer obituary? He can watch the scrounging and

gouging, he can hear the shouts of exultation, the moans of the gravely wounded, and meanwhile he feels secure; nobody will attack him from ambush.

Old age can also be a time of ennobling activity, as we are reminded by Tennyson. In "Ulysses," he wrote:

> Old age hath yet his honor and his toil;
> Death closes all; but something ere the end,
> Some work of noble note, may yet be done,
> Not unbecoming men that strove with gods.

He wrote that at 33, but let it guide his life for half a century more, and he published *Demeter and Other Poems* in 1889 at the age of 80.

These reminders of the possibilities for tranquility and accomplishment are important to keep in mind; they are useful antidotes to an overly pessimistic view. But they are not the whole story either. For there are both social and physical causes of the problems of the aged. Even in a utopian community, in which the social problems have been overcome, at times a sanguine view is out of place.

I think here of the contrast between my father in his early eighties and my grandmother, who died at 97. My father practiced law in Boston for nearly sixty years. In his late seventies and early eighties, he didn't put in quite a full week, but to the end he was still sprightly in his bow tie and as clever as they come. He was at work in his office on Beacon Street on Monday, February 22, 1988. On Tuesday, feeling unwell and suspecting that he was getting a fairly routine respiratory infection, he stayed home. That night he was taken to Beth Israel Hospital, where he died the following day at the age of eighty-two.

My grandmother, toward the end, had periods of lucidity with diminishing frequency. She lived in a world barely larger than her little space in a nursing home, uncomfortable much of the time, with little sense of herself or her circumstances. She had, close at hand, superbly capable medical care—also at Boston's Beth Israel, and she was saved by emergency medical care, including surgery, several times in her final years. At the time, I could easily imagine sending her a birthday card a decade or two later—though she was already long past being able to read one.

I'm not at all sure how we ought to respond to cases of that sort. Their numbers are increasing very rapidly—and further advances in life-sustaining technology may give the phrase "long term" an entirely new kind of impact as that technology enables the very old and very ill to remain very ill and become very much older. We should be equally interested in the role that technology can play in affecting the quality of the lives it helps to sustain.

Following rounds, I walk along the hospital corridor with a few of the physicians. We chat about the growing costs of medical care—about the constant use of tests and how quickly it runs the bill up. Once again, I hear mention of a notorious Mrs. T, who seems to be something of a legend in the hospital. I ask who she is, how long she has been in the hospital. A resident replies, "I don't know. She was here when I came last year. You ought to go see her."

Mrs. T is in the Pulmonary Intensive Care Unit. The staff on the unit are happy to tell me about her. Ninety-three years old now, she was admitted as an in-patient well over a year ago, and has had two birthdays in the hospital since then. Frail and very ill, she is dependent on a respirator. Unstable for many months, she eventually responded to treatment to the extent that her condition stabilized, and she has been stable now for several months. She can't get better, but with aggressive medical support, she doesn't get worse.

She has long since exhausted her Medicare benefits, and Medicaid in any case only covers 56% of costs. Her hospital bill approaches half a million dollars, which everyone knows will never be paid.

I ask a physician why she is kept here, why she can't be moved to a long-term care facility. He explains that there are just two chronic care hospitals in the area that have the capabilities to care for her, and the waiting lists are one to two years long. The problem is that such places provide very good patient maintenance, and so there is low turnover. Nobody wants to get into or expand the long-term chronic care business, he says, because it is poorly paid and there's so little psychological payoff. So Mrs. T stays here. There's nothing else to do with her.

It sounds to me like a clear case of overtreatment—of providing sophisticated medical intervention because it is possible, not because it is beneficial. How can such a life be worth sustaining at considerable effort and great cost? But I want to see for myself.

I enter the room accompanied by a doctor and a nurse. Mrs. T sits in a chair, staring at a television set. A daytime soap opera is playing. The nurse bends over and calls Mrs. T, who slowly turns her head toward us. A tube from the respirator enters her throat; she cannot speak. But she smiles faintly, and nods to me as we are introduced. So I realize that there is some cognition present. She turns back toward the television set.

"Mrs. T," I ask, "do you watch this every day?" She turns to me again, and nods affirmatively. "Suppose I change the channel to another program. Would that be all right?" Her eyes widen; she shakes her head negatively with such vigor that I fear she will shake loose her respirator tube!

"All right," I reassure her, "we'll leave it alone."

So there is definitely someone home. She cares about the world she watches on television; the plight of the players sustains her interest, and her curiosity carries her forward from one day to the next. She is living a life that has meaning for her, however empty it may seem to others.

Outside the room, I ask what her DNR status is. There is no DNR order for her, I learn; her daughter has declined to approve it. And, anyway, Mrs. T has been asked from time to time what her own wishes are. The doctor tells me of his conversation with her about her situation. After reviewing her condition and prognosis with her, he had said, "Now, you know Mrs. T, at your age and in your condition, it is possible that one day your heart may just stop. If that happens, how do you want us to act?"

Silently mouthing the words, she gave her unmistakable reply. "You start it."

In a simpler time, neither the television that sustains Mrs. T's interest nor the respirator that sustains her life existed. Now, technology of all sorts surrounds us. We use it in obvious ways to sustain the lives of the frail elderly. But I wonder how much more it could do to sustain their interest in life, as well, than enabling them to follow soap operas.

The availability of better technology to facilitate daily living for the very old is largely a function of market phenomena. What is already developed is not widely enough known or distributed, but the situation may improve as the relevant market increases. If the impaired elderly are to benefit from life-facilitating technologies, we must make them known to those whom they can help, and reduce the economic barriers that inhibit their use.

In addition to its obvious contributions to medical intervention, technology facilitates daily living for the elderly in many ways with such products as motorized wheelchairs, hearing aids, prosthetic devices, and the like. Technology can also provide more effective communication, for example, through telephones with volume amplification or enlarged numbers.

Sometimes, sophisticated communication systems make a vital difference, as with "Lifeline" systems that link a patient's home to the emergency room of a nearby hospital. Such systems function at more than 1000 hospitals; in some cases the patient's "help" button has a timed backup unit that will automatically summon help if the patient does not reset the timer on schedule.

Finally, technology can enrich the quality of daily life; the video cassette recorder that allows the house-bound to see films of their own choosing, rented by mail, is one example. Computers, too, may be central to this category.

Computers help the elderly lead safer and more healthful lives in various ways; examples include devices to monitor the home environment and programs to provide dietary analysis and menu planning. Again, it is largely a question of cost and distribution—in addition to some psychological barriers to their acceptance.

Medical applications of computer technology to the treatment of the elderly include aids to sensory perception, electronic prosthetic devices, and computer-aided diagnostic techniques—some of which are quite imaginative. For example, University of Texas neurologists use computers to monitor the video game performance of patients with Parkinson's disease; the results reveal disease progression and treatment effectiveness. With regard to life-enhancing technologies, I suspect we have not yet scratched the surface, however. This is the possibility that intrigues me the most.

A television advertisement some years ago showed a gleeful three-year-old enthralled at the family computer as his father dutifully prepared him for life in the information age. There's a strong suggestion that to deny any child a computer is a modern form of child abuse or at least a cruel cultural deprivation. Responsible parents have brought home computers by the millions. All over the country, kids are packed off to computer camps each summer, so they won't be left behind as the twenty-first century sweeps in on us. And school boards across the land agonize about how to acknowledge the computer age in their curricular planning and how to cope with the consequent budgetary demands.

Many adults still stand in horrified awe of the teen-age wizards who roam almost at will around other peoples' electronic memories. Fast fortunes are made by programming protégés, whose inventiveness can leave their elders dazzled. Troubled commentators ask what all this means for the future—what it portends for relationships between youth and adults, for the development of moral integrity, for interpersonal relationships, for our sense of what it means to be a human. We have entered the age of the computer, and the computer, it seems, belongs to the young.

At the same time, we recognize a wholesale change in the fabric of American society as the population ages. No longer is contemporary culture dominated by the hawkers of "the Pepsi generation." The Medicare and social security systems will strain under the pressure, and the requisite social adjustments will pose many new challenges. The future, it seems, belongs to the mature— with a substantial piece of it belonging to the very elderly.

These two aspects of contemporary life are a natural match. Computers have remarkable potential to enhance the lives of the aging, yet that potential has hardly been noticed within the computer industry. Perhaps the problem is that market surveys haven't shown a commercial potential great enough to motivate investment in such prospects. But if the demographers are right, that will surely change.

A small number of older citizens—a few in their 90s—have turned to programming as a hobby, or in pursuit of a post-retirement career. In May 1984, *Infoworld* reported that the Little House Senior Adults Community Center in Menlo Park, California, has an active computer club and an expanding enrollment in its computer classes. My concern, however, is neither with medical applications, nor with the ways in which well-functioning, mobile people can do, after retirement, what the rest of us can do with computers. I am intrigued instead by the special informational needs that computers can help meet to enhance the lives of people of great longevity, whose functional abilities are diminished in various ways and whose mobility is restricted—people of the sort I met in the Chelsea Nursing Home.

Some people scorn the idea of great longevity. (I don't mean immortality; I just mean living a very long time.) But I'm all for it. What motivates me is largely *curiosity.* I want to stay alive as long as I can, to see what happens—possibly even long enough to see the Boston Red Sox win the World Series. Many elderly people, physically debilitated in various ways, nonetheless delight in the spectacle of the unfolding of events. There's good news and bad news, to be sure, but all in all, it's quite a show.

Life for the very old, especially when accompanied by serious illness, lacks the diversity of earlier years. It becomes dominated by the basic needs of physical survival and by behavior focused centrally on the handling of information—be it watching a soap opera (as Mrs. T did each day), talking with friends or health care workers, keeping up with the news, providing an oral history within the family, reading Aristotle (as Oliver Wendell Holmes is said to have done on his deathbed in his 90s), or simply enjoying the pleasures of reminiscing. New information-processing technology could be put to much better use in serving these interests, helping elderly people maintain active and interested minds. Nothing is more crucial to the quality of their lives in their declining years.

At the Hebrew Home of Greater Washington, Shulamith Weisman conducted a pilot project in 1982, providing modified computer games for 50 frail, elderly residents whose average age was 85. This unstaffed, unfunded project was made possible by a five-month loan of an Apple Computer from the Apple Corporation and by the donated efforts of a local programmer, who adapted the software of four commercial games to make them suited to the setting. Primarily, he increased the size of visual images and reduced the pace of the action to allow for slower response times. The residents seemed well pleased with the project; one observed, "If the whole world is going crazy over computer games, why shouldn't we get in on the fun?" Ms. Weisman found the experiment to have intriguing results in increased vitality of and interaction among the residents, and concluded that "The computer industry should be made aware of the potential of a market of elderly consumers. It may then be encouraged to research the needs of this ever growing segment of society." ("Computer Games for the Frail Elderly," *The Gerontologist*, v. 23, no. 4, 1983). There is no evidence that the industry has noticed, however.

But I don't have in mind simply putting computer games in nursing homes. Books and magazines could be made available at terminals on demand, with the text appearing in whatever size print and intensity of brightness and contrast are best suited to the individual reader. Vidoetex systems, which link a terminal with information services, communication networks, and even travel and purchasing arrangements, provide some of the resources that would serve such a purpose, although new programs would have to be written to allow user adjustments that compensate for sensory deficits. Some hardware modifications might be needed as well, such as enlarged keyboards, designed not for speed, but for users who have little manual dexterity, yet much patience.

Friends in different locations could play chess or checkers, or otherwise interact, by using interconnected terminals. That will require the establishment of appropriate networks, perhaps linking community centers with one another and with nursing homes, so that residents can maintain social interaction with friends with different degrees of independence and mobility. People of any age who recognize the value of learning as an activity, apart from practical benefits it may foster, could enjoy educational programs that match their interests, level of sophistication, and mobility. That will require access by the elderly to educational software. A modest, but sustained investment in research and development would surely lead to beneficial products in the near future. Problems of cost, allocation, training, and maintenance will attend the development of any such products, but I see no reason to consider them unsolvable.

A few years ago in San Francisco, a psychiatrist proposed the establishment of a nonprofit firm devoted to developing applications of information technology for the elderly—to explore the kinds of hardware and software that meet the needs of the elderly, and then introduce computer applications into senior centers, seeking to stimulate social interaction and enhance self-esteem and general psychological wellbeing. Such activities could lead to a product line including specially designed recreational and informational software, modified hardware packages, instructional support to facilitate the introduction of the products, and an on-line informational network tailored to the needs of the elderly and the centers that serve them.

In 1981, some of these issues were addressed in a symposium at Case Western Reserve University. In the proceedings of that conference (*Communications Technology and the Elderly*, ed. Dunkle, Haug, and Rosenberg, Springer Publishing Co., 1984) R. J. Nelson warned of the dangers of infatuation with technology as a remedy for the social isolation of elderly people. "Human-to-machine conversation . . . is liable to degrade the quality of human existence, not enhance it, especially for the elderly," he cautioned. To appreciate the reality of that risk, one need only reflect on the irresponsible and intellectually stultifying way television sets have been used by many harried parents as an easy remedy for some of the demands of caring for their children.

Computer terminals should never substitute for sustained, compassionate, human contact with the very old. As Walter A. Rosenblith emphasized in the keynote address at the symposium, "Terminals themselves can generate new forms of loneliness . . . it is the interaction with fellow humans that seems to bring out in most of us optimal utilization of our information processing capacities." But the risks need not deter us from a prudent pursuit of the gains that could result from supplementing human contact with judicious use of technology. Computer applications that can enrich the lives of the elderly will be a sound investment in the future.

Nelson wisely urged that such developments should proceed

with "input at the planning and design stages from older individuals themselves." The necessary collaboration can take place on a small scale, by means of ad hoc arrangements between fledgling companies and institutions and agencies in their vicinity involved in the care of the elderly. It can also proceed on a large scale, through cooperative ventures jointly undertaken by major computer and software companies and such national organizations as the American Association of Retired Persons and the various other associations dedicated to advocating and serving the interests of the aged.

For society, this may indeed be the information age. But for each of us, advanced years are the information age. It is time to begin applying all that we know about information technology to the interests and needs of the elderly. We're not that far behind them.

That, however, is just a prudential reason to favor greater investment now in the conditions of life of the elderly; it is an investment that may later pay direct personal dividends to us in our own final years. But the case does not rest purely on such prudential reasoning. Generosity toward the aged is obligatory for other reasons, based on considerations of respect and entitlement that do not depend on our own future interests. Yet how do we balance that generosity against our own interests and our sense of obligation to our children and future generations? How do we draw that line? This issue is at the center of vigorous current debate about the costs of health care for the very ill, very old.

Three perspectives may help clarify the moral underpinnings of our contemporary deliberations about these matters and about the conflicting values they involve. The first is the familiar consequentialist perspective, according to which the right thing to do is whatever produces the best consequences—as judged against some standard of what counts as a good consequence. Usually the measure is taken to be human happiness, so that right actions are those that maximize happiness and minimize suffering. That view, exemplified by the utilitarianism of John Stuart Mill, has been the dominant influence in our moral thought and our public policy debates for the last hundred years.

The utilitarian mandate to produce the greatest good for the greatest number supports our inclinations to beneficence. It offers an explanation of why we should do good for others, even absent their request that we do so. But it is rife with difficulties, for there seem to be deep conflicts between the utilitarian concern with social interests, on the one hand, and the need to protect individual rights, on the other. Even if more total human happiness would be produced by simply abandoning an aged and costly ancestor to whom we have clear commitments, it is unlikely that we would have any right to do so.

Despite such problems inherent in consequentialist moral thought, most policy justifications are cast in precisely these terms. Policymakers especially focus on the outcomes of the choices before them, and cost-benefit analysis reflects the belief that a consideration of the probable consequences ought to determine what we do.

The consequentialist view of morality does not go unchallenged. There is another tradition of moral thought, going back at least to the Ten Commandments, according to which consequences are not the determinants of the moral quality of our actions. Rather, some actions are held to be morally required, and others forbidden, because of the kinds of actions they are. Thus, we have a commandment that instructs: Honor thy father and mother. It does not say: Honor thy father and mother, unless it turns out that more human happiness will result from your doing otherwise. Such commandments do not have escape clauses or footnotes restricting their range of applicability. They enjoin us to look not to the future, to what the consequences of our action will probably be, but rather to the actions themselves or to the commitments we have, based on past actions and relationships. The continued care of Mrs. T, for example, was never defended in the hospital on the basis of any analysis of costs versus benefits. Her treatment was sustained in the conviction that it was an obligation of caring in the context of the hospital and its inherent values and traditions—an obligation that was not dispelled even by the very high costs.

The leading philosophical proponent of such nonconsequentialist morality was Immanuel Kant, an eighteenth-century philosopher who held that respect for persons as autonomous rational agents lies at the core of morality. He is perhaps best known for the "categorical imperative," the most useful version of which states that one ought never to treat others as means only, but should always respect them as ends unto themselves. Such a principle precludes slavery, punishment of the innocent, and other forms of exploitation no matter what the potential societal benefits might be. These acts are wrong because of the kinds of acts they are, and one therefore need not even inquire into their consequences.

But this perspective, too, is laden with difficulties. First, it fails to guide us through many kinds of moral conflict, including those all too common situations in which the moral rules we try to follow are in conflict with one another. Second, this perspective ignores the potentially devastating social costs of absolute compliance with its moral strictures.

Literally to maximize the autonomy of those in long-term care would require massive investments that might be disastrous for other needs such as education, public health, housing programs, and the like. Are we really to exclude all thought of such matters from our deliberations? Are we really willing to invest an unlimited amount of the national wealth in the care of the very ill, very old?

A more recent perspective was provided by John Rawls in *A Theory of Justice* (1971)—a classic in its own time. Many people refer to that work, although far fewer have read it. That is no surprise; it has 87 sections, rough going all the way. One of its central ideas is a particularly useful heuristic here, however.

Imagine—this is farfetched, but helpful—that you and I, and several others, have been appointed to a commission empowered by the government to determine a definitive policy for the long-term care of the very ill, very old. We are strictly obliged to complete our task promptly, come what may. We are drafting our report one evening when a terrible storm raises the building we are in right above the clouds. After the storm, the building has settled gently back down, and we can resume our discussion. But we are cut off without any links to the outside world, and there is a new problem now.

We've spun around so much that a strange sort of selective amnesia afflicts us all. We recall all that we knew about that outside world—a lot of physics, sociology, economics, history, medicine, and all the rest. Yet we find ourselves utterly devoid of any specific knowledge about ourselves. We just can't remember who we are, or what. There's a faint buzzing in our ears that makes all voices sound alike to us, regardless of age or sex. And our vision is a bit blurred, so although we can see one another, we can't make any distinctions among people—ourselves included. It will go away eventually, of course; this veil of ignorance about ourselves will lift. Meanwhile, we must get on with the conversation; we must decide what to do about long-term care. (A hint of what such a conversation might be like occurs when one participates in a conference call involving several people whom one does not know.)

Rawls holds that the principles of a just society are those that would be mutually acceptable to rational persons negotiating under just such a veil of ignorance. But our agenda is more restricted; we need only decide on a policy for long-term care.

As we discuss the matter, we realize that certain policies will benefit some persons to the disadvantage of others. Investing half the national wealth in the care of those over 85 will do very nicely for them, but will be disastrous for those just approaching adulthood. How do you vote on such a policy, even assuming that you are interested merely in doing as well for yourself as you can? That will depend, among other things, on your age. If you are 20, you'll be against it. If you are 85, you may think it just fine.

Here is where the veil of ignorance has its effect. Since you know nothing that will distinguish you from anyone else, you have no idea of your own age. So you are required by the logic of the situation to favor only those policies that will be fair to you no matter who or what you turn out to be when the veil lifts—for example, whether you are an elderly patient, a nursing home administrator, a healthy young taxpayer, or a poor student struggling to pay for your education.

You will have to ask a different question from those asked either by the Kantian or by the utilitarian: What sort of community can I reasonably endorse, not knowing where I will fit into it? Not knowing whether I will be a recipient of long-term care, a provider of such care, or simply a taxpayer supporting such care—how do I want such matters to be handled? Asking that question can help one transcend the parochialism of one's own perspective, and gain a broader sense of what is fair and just.

The question of what is a just and reasonable social policy for the care of the elderly is treated in two recent, influential works by philosophers, Norman Daniels' *Am I My Parents Keeper: An*

Essay on Justice Between the Young and the Old, and Daniel Callahan's widely debated *Setting Limits: Medical Goals in an Aging Society.* Both books challenge the notion that we should provide to the very old and very ill whatever care might benefit them; what prompts that challenge is the recognition that in an era of high-technology health care, we cannot possibly pay the bill for such unlimited care delivered to an expanding population.

Where medical intervention saves a life that would otherwise be lost, the result is a patient instead of a body—a patient who may then need long-term care. Our successes in medicine thus increase the demand for medical care, instead of saturating it, and contribute to that expanding population.

Consider Barney Clark, the first recipient of a totally implantable artificial heart—an example chosen just to illustrate the new sense of "long term" that we must begin to ponder. As I wrote in 1983 (*The Los Angeles Times*, January 14, p.11), shortly before he died,

> We're all rooting for Barney Clark—that medical pioneer, man of courage, and symbol of our desire to defeat our own mortality. I do admire him and wish him well; I'd love to learn one day that his life is again robust and full, and worth the awesome price he has paid to sustain it.
>
> But there is something deeply troubling as I contemplate his future and ours. Assume that, as we all hope, his artificial heart keeps working indefinitely without any further difficulty, and that he adjusts to his resulting life as well as can reasonably be hoped. The day will come all the same when something else will go awry. Even now, he has had some spells of kidney insufficiency; perhaps it will be the kidneys that are next to go.
>
> Imagine that you are one of Barney Clark's doctors on that fateful day. Do you turn your back on this triumph of modern medical skill, and condemn him to the death that has been forestalled so dramatically? Or do you send him on to the dialysis unit, where kidney failure is just a problem to be solved, not a fatal deficiency?
>
> The British Health Service does not typically dialyze patients Clark's age; that helps to keep a lid on their national medical bill. But you're not likely to let our Barney go like that, just to save the cost. Not after the emotional, intellectual, and financial investments that have already been made.

Anyway, we don't like the idea of making vital decisions on the basis of what the bill will be. We have a national policy of providing dialysis to anyone whose life can be saved that way. We're certainly not going to discriminate against Clark just because he has a mechanical heart. So off he goes to the dialysis unit, where a mechanical kidney does the trick.

Twenty years ago, with a prescience not unusual for him, Kurt Vonnegut wrote a little play called *Fortitude*. Sylvia, the heroine, has been saved from death by modern medical technology. She's got a mechanical heart and she's on dialysis. She's had her liver replaced by a newly developed artificial one. Her pancreas was custom made. In fact, by the time we meet her, the only original equipment that is left is her head—connected to a roomful of devices, monitors, and controls. Now *that's* medical progress! Lucky for her she's the widow of a billionaire.

I don't mean to suggest that we should simply put on the brakes and stop developing or applying advances in medical technology. But we do need to think very hard about the road ahead. I'd dialyze Barney Clark, too, if that's what he wanted. But I worry about how much of this sort of thing is for the best.

In principle, we can greatly reduce the costs of dialysis through an increased public awareness of the need to donate transplantable kidneys. And perhaps one day the artificial heart will be small, reliable, and of moderate cost. But something else—a liver or a pancreas—will then capture our attention in the front ranks of medicine's inexorable march forward. And the cost will matter, like it or not.

We now spend 10% [a figure that in 1987 was more than 11%] of the Gross National Product on health care—nearly 300 billion dollars a year [which rose to more than $500 billion in 1987, the most recent year for which figures are available from the Health Care Financing Administration]. There is no possibility of saturating the market, of meeting the demand. The more success we have, the more demand we sustain—just as the success of the Jarvik 7 heart sustains Barney Clark as a health care consumer.

I don't know what the answer is to the problem of deciding how much is enough, but I do know it is time to start looking for it. Modern medicine is in its adolescence—delighted and awed by the rush of new powers that have come upon it almost overnight, and yet not old enough to have developed a seasoned, mature sense of just how to use those dazzling, irresistible, frightening, and almost mysterious abilities.

That maturity of judgment won't come easily, and it probably won't come soon. Maybe it will take a few hundred years to develop. And maybe we'll be around to see it when it does. Or, at least, maybe our heads will be.

In recent years, there have been many changes in health care. The nation has turned away from the totally implantable artificial heart (although Robert Jarvik continues to work on its refinement with private funding) in favor of improving the LVAD—the left ventricular assist device; the percentage of our GNP spent on health care has climbed even higher; AIDS has captured the medical spotlight; the powers of genetic intervention have developed further, we face the prospect of successful mapping of the complete human genome; and so on. But the same basic problems remain. Whereas just a few decades ago it was rare for anyone to be very old and very ill for very long, now it is a frequent outcome of the use of our new medical powers.

An elderly woman in the hospital has circulatory problems, among others. The attending physician gently feels her feet and ankles, then asks, "Do you like it better when it's warm or cool?" She shrugs her shoulders. He asks again, "What do you like best?"

"I like it best," she replies, "when it's just right."

Another woman has severe respiratory distress. "How's your breathing this morning?" the doctor asks.

"A little," she answers.

"A little better or a little worse?"

"A little breathing," she explains.

.7.
. . .

AT THE END
OF LIFE

The hospital never stops. At any hour of the day or night, people come and go, trudging through their routine chores, living out their private dramas, wrestling with their fears, reacting to the unexpected. To the patient, everyone else is a visitor, the doctor no less than family or friends. To the private practitioner, the hospital is the most sophisticated of all medical resources, a complex technology always available to aid a patient in distress. To the interns and residents—the house officers—it becomes nearly the world, as the long hours and heavy demands of their lives as physicians in training leave little time or energy for anything beyond the hospital's walls.

It is 4:45 A.M.; I have been asleep for about two and a half hours on the lower bunk of a stark, narrow cell containing only the bunks, two metal lockers, a small nightstand, and a telephone. Light and noise flow in from the corridor, but with no more effect on me than on Arthur, asleep on the upper bunk with the telephone, its cord stretched to the limit, inches from his head. I have no dreams, no recollections of the depressing drabness of the room, no awareness of the narrow bunk or thin, stiff pillow.

Suddenly, Arthur grabs the telephone on the first ring, emitting some syllable faintly suggestive of reluctantly emerging consciousness. He listens for about two seconds, and in two seconds more is at the door, shifting into high gear. "What have we got?" I ask, groping for my shoes. Arthur, who had never removed his, replies over his shoulder, "Arrest on 7," and is halfway down the hall as I bolt through the door in pursuit.

By the time we get to the scene of the cardiac arrest, a dozen people surround the patient. The medical resident is choreographing a resuscitation effort. Arthur, an intern, leaps into the battle. In a matter of minutes, tubes of diverse kinds are threaded into various places—one into the neck, another into an arm, a third into the lungs. The intermittent compression of the patient's chest by the rescue team lends a steady beat to the visual scene; various monitors add their sights and sounds to the spectacle.

I drop back from the center of action, not wanting to intrude on this struggle against death. The patient, of whom I have a clear view, is an older woman lying large, pale, and unresponding at the center of the commotion. I wonder whether she has ever before been the focus of so much attention, whether in her conscious life there have ever been moments when so many people have acted so single-mindedly in her behalf. But she cannot enjoy this attention; I learn that she has pervasive, end-stage cancer—that she has been in a coma for several days prior to the cardiac arrest, responsive only to deep pain stimulus. I wonder what the point can be of this tour de force of medical power; the intern answers my unspoken question, softly grumbling, "There's no point to this at all." But his participation in the effort is uncompromising.

I notice an empty bed near the door; we are in 765, a semiprivate room, and the action is around the bed near the window. There are rumpled linens on the empty bed; I look around for its occupant. Like the others on the scene, I want to be of help, to do something useful. But I am neither doctor nor nurse; at most I can hope to stay out of the way.

The count in the room is now sixteen, and it is getting crowded. I slip into the hall and look around. At the far end of the corridor a woman stands, wearing a bathrobe, looking confused. I ask a nurse about the roommate of the dying patient. She replies, "We try to get them out if we can. It can be pretty upsetting to them. I told her she could go to the solarium."

"Where is transport? Did you call them?" One of the doctors is eager to get a blood gas report, but the sample has not yet gone down for analysis. The runner who is to take it to the lab has been *called, but is nowhere to be seen. A nurse calls again, complaining of the delay.*

I walk past three or four rooms to the woman standing at the end of the hall and ask if she is the displaced patient. She is, and volunteers that she has been advised to go to the solarium. I tell her it's a good idea and walk along with her, just a few steps, into the comfortably furnished unoccupied room. I look out through the expanse of glass at the panorama of a city, peacefully aglow with the first light of a new day. It is a beautiful scene, but Mrs. A doesn't notice it. She settles tiredly into a chair, and looks quizzically at me. "Has anyone told you what's going on?" I ask. "No," she replies, "but it's Mrs. M. I hope she makes it. I don't even know her."

"They're doing what they can," I assure her. "But there are a lot of people in the room, and it's very crowded and noisy. I'm sure you'll be more comfortable here." She smiles at me and, comforted, says "Thank you, Doctor."

"I'm just an observer," I answer, feeling a bit out of place, but not even slightly tempted to explain my presence. As I walk back to the patient's room, I think of how terrifying it must be to be awakened by the sudden eruption of a mortal crisis a few feet from one's bed and to find oneself moments later at the end of the hall entirely alone with one's own intimations of mortality accentuated so abruptly.

Back in 765, Mrs. M has begun to respond. Against the odds, the resuscitation is succeeding. Her heart is beating once again. Snatched back from the jaws of death, hers is a life saved by dazzling intervention. She is, of course, still in a coma, and is now on a respirator. But she is stable for the moment, and the crowd around her begins to shrink.

I ask the resident if it would be appropriate for me to talk to the evicted roommate, to tell her what the fuss has been about. He encourages me, so I return to the solarium and give Mrs. A a brief summary of the situation. She nods appreciatively; a nurse comes in and sits down with us. She takes over where I have left off, now turning her attention to Mrs. A's concerns. I head back to 765.

In the corridor, the conversation turns to Mrs. M's prognosis; it is agreed that she has no significant chance of meaningful recovery. Now that she is stable, however, she must go to the coronary intensive care unit where her vital functions can be monitored continuously. So a team of six slides her from her bed onto a cart, and amidst her medical entourage, she is wheeled toward the elevators that take her down to the fifth floor. Along the way, the doctors and nurses pursue a question they raised as the rescue effort began: why resuscitate this woman?

At one level, the answer is clear. She arrested, and when a patient arrests, the response follows automatically, for better or worse, unless there is a DNR order in the patient's medical chart. For Mrs. M the chart leaves no room for doubt; a note from the attending physician reports that he has raised the question with her children and that they are adamant in both their refusal to approve of DNR status and their insistence that everything possible be done for their mother. So the hospital staff had no choice within the confines of the hospital's policy.

She will likely arrest again. There is a flurry of telephone activity. The resident calls the attending doctor at home, then calls one of the daughters. With the attending doctor's approval, the resident gently raises the question of what should be done if there is another arrest. He arranges to meet the daughter later, in the intensive care unit.

The crowd of seven has dispersed; Mrs. M is now in the ICU. There is no roommate here, no window to the outer world. She lies on her bed, comprehending nothing, conscious of nothing, never to be conscious again. But we are exquisitely conscious of her—of every available detail of the fluids and gases and pressures and rhythms of her faltering physiology. Here, she will remain, under constant scrutiny, until some new turn of events signals the start of the next round.

It is after six now. I am totally tired, but there is no point in going back to the "on-call" room. It is too late to get any real sleep, and, anyway, I am not sleepy. My head spins with unanswered questions. Have I just witnessed an example of medical progress, of a medical nightmare, or of both? How do these young doctors and nurses maintain their motivation in the face of such demanding tasks that offer so little gratification in return? Why was there no DNR order for this hopeless, dying woman? When should there be such orders? Mrs. M's children wanted everything possible done for her. Have I just seen something done for her or to her?

Should her physician have been more assertive with her children in recommending a DNR order? Why did the family want the futile struggle to continue? Should the wishes of family members always be respected, no matter how strongly the medical staff disagrees? What if the family members disagree among themselves?

Perhaps I am overreacting to the futility of what I have seen. A more liberal use of DNR orders might carry worse costs than the occasional bit of futility. After all, Mrs. M was past minding what was done for or to her. She can't really be thought of as a victim. Yet it is horrible to contemplate the same sort of end: hopelessly past sentience, splayed out naked on a bed, being worked on by a bunch of young doctors who would derive much more benefit from an extra hour's sleep than I could possibly derive from them.

Funny how my mind keeps returning to the idea of sleep. I'll have to sort out all these questions later, when I've had some.

I wander back to my office in the hospital. I have promised to review a draft before leaving at noon for a meeting in New York. But I have a meeting at nine in OBGYN, and at eleven there will be a discussion about a patient judged mentally competent and then admitted to the hospital over her objections and treated despite her protests. I certainly want to participate in that. So I'd best do the draft at once, before dashing back to my apartment to pack for New York.

I make several suggestions on the draft, leave the office, and walk out to the hospital garage. I have been in my clothes for twenty-four hours, and feel as rumpled as they look. I am tempted to go home and sleep until it is time to head for the airport. But I recall that Arthur must soon be back on the medical unit for the start of a new day, caring for patients despite his fatigue, teaching and learning together with the medical students, the residents, and the senior physicians. The thought shames me into resolving to be on time for my meeting at nine.

I pull out of the garage, into the waking city, heading for the apartment and the shower.

There was a time, long past, when saving lives whenever possible was uncontroversial. Now we can sometimes save the lives of patients whose lives are so diminished and whose prospects are so poor that no good purpose can be served by doing so.

Recognizing that fact is easy for most people. But it is hard to become clear about what follows from that recognition. At least the practice of striving always to save lives eliminates the need to make painful distinctions among patients, drawing a line that classifies some as worth saving and others not.

We would avoid those decisions if we could, but there are too many pressures to allow us that comfortable escape. They come from many directions. The most compelling pressure is our concern for the interests of patients; we realize that some patients may be harmed rather than helped by life-sustaining treatment.

This is most clearly the case when a terminally ill patient is close to death, is suffering, and then is threatened by infection or cardiac arrest. In the days before antibiotics and sophisticated resuscitative techniques, such a patient's ordeal would then end. Now it can be prolonged, so that some patients fear a medical response to their decline as an aggravation of their distress, rather than looking to medical care with hope as a source of comfort. Sometimes, they seek to protect themselves in advance against unwanted medical treatment they may be unable later to ward off; this they may do by expressing their views to family or physician, or through such devices as the "living will"—an oddly named, written record of a person's objection to being provided with medical treatment that is death-prolonging more than life-sustaining. (It is sometimes, more suitably, called an "advance directive.") Some hospitals now call this possibility to the attention of the communities they serve, making sample declarations available and advising that such documents be kept in a safe place and be made known to "a person's family, physician, and legal counsel."

It is also possible in most states to designate a health care proxy empowered to exercise authoritative discretion in a patient's behalf if the patient is unable to function competently. Many states and the District of Columbia have passed such legislation, others have achieved the same result by amending the provisions regarding durable powers of attorney so that such powers may be extended to cover health care decisions, and more have modified their "living will" statutes to provide for the delegation of decision-making powers to others for a broader range of treatment decisions than just those that concern life-sustaining treatment.

The Health Care Proxy bill in New York, however, as proposed by the New York State Task Force on Life and the Law (a body appointed by and advisory to the Governor, and chaired by the Commissioner of Health), did not pass when it was considered in 1989. Although such legislation is favored by a broad public consensus and was supported by many diverse organizations, there remained some concern in the legislature about its long-term impact. Despite such concerns, the bill was finally passed on July 1, 1990, just after an important United States Supreme Court decision in the matter of Cruzan.

At issue was one of the most difficult challenges to have emerged in the last few years, the question of the conditions under which it is appropriate to withdraw artificial nutrition and hydration from a patient who is not terminally ill. Such cases have yielded mixed results in state courts, and the Supreme Court, in the Cruzan case, upheld the Missouri law that restricts the rights of family members to direct the withdrawal of such treatment in the absence of written evidence of the patient's wishes that is clear and compelling. The concern of some disputants is that an unrestricted health care proxy could favor the withdrawal of artificial nutrition and hydration in the case of an irreversibly comatose patient, and the hold that there is a legitimate public interest in preventing such outcomes no matter what the patient would have wanted.

The political resistance in New York had the support of at least one conservative religious leader. Cardinal John J. O'Connor, writhing in *Catholic New York* (July 20, 1989), explained why he refrained from supporting the bill, affirming that any concern for the relief of human suffering should be tempered by a respect for what he calls the "tremendous potential of suffering":

A frightening number of people are being condemned to death by the courts, at the request of loved ones or "proxies," or by their own personal requests. The reason: They are suffering "needlessly"; their lives are "useless"; they are terminally ill, or comatose, or "have nothing to live for." What an enormous difference it could make to such patients or to those acting on their behalf, if they understood the power of suffering. . . . I believe that a bill *could* be fashioned that would prohibit unconditional withdrawal of nutrition and hydration no matter *who* ordered or requested it. . . . I believe a bill is possible that will once and for all make clear that not even the patient has ultimate control over his or her own life. . . . In the meanwhile, those suffering unto death merit our thanking them for their testimony to life—and for helping us save our souls.*

Some experience of suffering undoubtedly enhances one's understanding of the suffering of others, and thereby empowers one to deal with them more empathetically. But the suffering of the dying lacks that prudential advantage. Whether the value of other suffering should outweigh personal autonomy, or whether considerations of the quality of life should have weight, are, in the last analysis, more a matter of basic value choice than of reasoned conclusion.

A plausible basis of concern about decisions to withdraw artificial nutrition and hydration is perhaps based on the recognition that two distinct tensions exist in the context of such decisions. First, there is the tension between our widely shared, generalized respect for life, and a specific concern about the quality of the life of the patient at issue. Most of us are willing to grant that in some circumstances, consideration of the quality of a person's life is more significant than the mere continuation of some level of biological functioning. But not all agree, and for those to whom such quality of life considerations are anathema, the withdrawal of life-sustaining interventions is hard to justify—especially when no case can be made that the intervention is simply the prolongation of a dying.

Second, there is the tension between our widely shared, general commitment to the primacy of the interests of the patient, and our concern in particular cases that the continued existence of the patient in a condition of total and uncomprehending dependency constitutes an undue burden on others, most usually the patient's family, as well as an affront to the values that the patient held when sentient. Here, too, most agree that it can be reasonable to give some weight to the impact on a family—just as most people would wish such factors to be respected in the event that they are

---

*For a critical exploration of this view of suffering, see William Nicholson's compelling drama *Shadowlands*.

the patient in question. And here, again, not all agree that such factors may safely or justly be considered.

In each of these tensions, the prevailing public sentiment favors a process that allows the lines between the conflicting values to be drawn flexibly, taking into account what is known about or is most probably true of the values of the patient, and giving some weight, as the patient would likely have favored, to the interests of others impacted by the patient's plight. A dissenting minority, however—sincere and influential, prefers to avoid the risks of excess by prohibiting such flexibility at the outset.

Even when a competent patient has clearly expressed an objection to receiving life-sustaining medical treatment, the possibility remains that it will be imposed. A few highly publicized cases, perhaps very atypical, nonetheless have fueled fears about that possibility. One such case is that of William Bartling, who in 1984 asked that his treatment in a California hospital be discontinued. He was terminally ill, deplored his painful life on a respirator, was declining inexorably, and knew it. The hospital took a firm position in favor of prolonging his life to the maximum possible extent despite his objections. He sought judicial relief; the hospital opposed him in that effort.

Thus the battle raged—the hospital fighting against death and Bartling fighting against the hospital. In the end, on appeal, the courts ruled in favor of Bartling's right to refuse life-sustaining treatment. But he never knew of that victory. He had declined beyond the point of sentience, and then died, before the case was concluded.

It is a well-established and widely regarded principle that to impose treatment on an unwilling patient is at least a tort for which the injured party can claim compensation, and such imposition of treatment may constitute a battery. The moral view is widely shared that due regard for the autonomy of persons requires respecting their rights as individuals to decline even what others correctly judge to be in their interests. Then how could the Bartling case have happened, and what does it suggest about modern hospital care?

Few of us will find the phrase "Doctor knows best" to be unfamiliar. Doctors must rank close to mothers and fathers in this regard. Of course, there are many things that doctors do know best, and how to prolong the life of a seriously ill patient is among them. There is also a deep and genuine commitment among physicians—the occasional medical rogue aside—to serving the interests of their patients. That commitment can lead to zealousness in defense of life, a zealousness that can distort the physician's judgment about just what is in the patient's interest. And, increasingly, there is the fear of legal jeopardy.

In the Bartling case, there is reason to believe that his physicians were willing to follow his wishes and remove him from the ventilator—but only with the approval of the hospital's administration. The administration was willing to approve, but only with clearance from the hospital's legal counsel. That clearance was not forthcoming, however. The primary commitment of a hospital's lawyer is typically to minimize that hospital's legal risk—a very different objective from that of serving the interests of the patients. In this case, the hospital's attorneys, because of confusion about the law, misunderstanding of legal precedents, and concern to protect the hospital maximally against prosecution and litigation, rendered advice that was directly contrary to the interests and expressed wishes of the patient, who paid the price in frustration and continued suffering. (See George Annas's "Prisoner in the ICU: The Tragedy of William Bartling," *The Hastings Center Report*, December 1984.)

The current complexity of health care decisions is thus compounded by the overlay of fear, suspicion, and self-protection that is a consequence of our overreliance on the courts as mechanisms of conflict resolution. Even when doctor, family, and patient agree about the appropriate course of action, there may be bureaucratic barriers to pursuing that course, and the patient's interests may not prevail. For that reason, it is all the more important that those interests be clearly perceived from the beginning.

No patient's interests should be assumed on the basis of generalizations or convention. That most patients want their lives prolonged was no reason to prolong Bartling's life. That physicians are most comfortable using their skills on the side of life is no reason, either. The lawyers' fear that legal action might flow from withdrawal of treatment is obviously no good reason. But when, and how, to call off the medical troops?

The Bartling case was comparatively easy. He knew his circumstances, expressed his preferences clearly and in a reasoned way, and was simply a victim of bad legal judgment distorting medical care. Now that the courts have found in his favor, it is somewhat less likely that future patients in such circumstances will endure the same fate. And even Bartling would have been spared that fate had he been in a less doctrinaire and more sensitive medical environment.

But one does not always have the luxury of clearly expressed patient preferences in situations of medical gravity.

I sit in my office, reading a roster of the hospital's administrative staff, trying to link the names with a dozen or two of the faces I have met in the last day. The phone rings; a neurosurgeon has heard that I am at the hospital and thinks I might be interested in a case he has just confronted. I meet him immediately in the surgical intensive care unit (SICU).

The patient, 82, otherwise in good health, has fallen down a flight of stairs, breaking his neck in two places. Rushed to the emergency room, he was taken directly to surgery, but little could be done. His life has been saved, but his spinal cord is severed near the base of his skull. He lies with his head in traction, motionless, silent, with only the pulsating of the respirator to suggest that he might be alive.

"He is permanently paralyzed, completely, from the neck down," the doctor tells me. "He can never breathe without the respirator. He will never be able to speak, because of the respirator tube and because he can't produce the breath necessary for speech."

I ask about his brain, about his cognitive functioning. "We don't have any idea. He doesn't respond. He may have severe brain damage. He may be terrified. His mind may be intact."

"What would you expect the natural course to be if you make no efforts beyond maximizing his comfort?" I inquire.

"It's hard to say. He'll get an infection, his heart will stop. In days, maybe weeks."

"And how long could you keep him alive?" The doctor confirms my hunch. "It's indeterminate. A long time. Months. Years, maybe."

The patient has no capacity to express his preferences, or anything else. At 82, if he regains significant sentience, he faces the prospect of confronting total dependency as a silent quadriplegic. What should he be told of his circumstances? Is it best that he survive? In a case like this, the family must speak for the patient. Their knowledge of him and their concern for him presumably combine to make them the best available advocates for his interests. But the family too has received a severe injury, and their distress clouds their perception and their judgment.

Is a DNR order appropriate here? How clear should the physician be in stating his own views to the family in the midst of their confusion and vulnerability? And what if the family wants "everything possible" to be done, as they so often do? Is that devotion or guilt at work? Is it an admirable tenacity or a denial of reality?

A nurse joins our discussion. She tells us that the patient will open his eyes and seems to look at her. But he does not respond in any meaningful way. Grasping at straws, I suggest the obvious. "Have you tried to get him to blink his eyes, as signals?" She has, he doesn't. But his skin is starting to break down in places because of the pressure and friction of contact with the bedding. A special space-age bed has been ordered for him from a company that rents such things to hospitals; he will float on a cushion of tiny, aerated plastic spheres. That will help with the effort to prevent the bedsores from becoming horrible.

Several hours later, I return to the SICU. A grandson is visiting the patient. The young man stands beside the bed, speaking loudly. "Grandpa, can you hear me? It's Ben. Open your eyes, Grandpa!" The old man opens his eyes. His head remains rigid but his eyes look to the left. He stares, expressionless, at the source of the sound. Ben moves around to the right of the bed and speaks again. The eyes shift to the right.

The grandson turns to the doctor and to me, and says, "He understands every word. I know he does."

"Can you blink your eyes for me Grandpa? Blink your eyes at me." There is no response.

It seemed to me that the patient understood nothing at all, that the movement of his eyes toward the source of the familiar voice was a fairly primitive or perhaps even random response, signifying almost nothing about his mental state. The grandson, I thought, was grasping at straws. That's a normal reaction to tragic events, of course, and not a reaction to be criticized. Still, if the perceptions of family members are distorted by false hopes, how can they make reasoned judgments about what is best to do?

It is possible, too, that my own perceptions were distorted by a false sense of hope. Knowing the man's physical plight, I suddenly realized, I didn't *want* him to regain his mental acuity. I thought it better for him never to understand the situation he was in, to worry about the ailing wife who had been dependent on him, or to suffer the frustrations of a life of total dependency without even the capacity to ask questions or express himself. Surely that would be as close an approximation to hell on earth as one could devise. So the grandson and I were each seeing what we preferred. But what followed for the patient's treatment? In particular, should he be made DNR?

Boston's Beth Israel was among the first (1981) to adopt a formal set of guidelines governing the writing of DNR orders. That policy, 4 1/2 pages set in type, became a model for policy statements and statutes in various places. It states clearly that the expressed wishes of a competent and accurately informed patient must be respected, and describes procedures designed to assure a cautious and reliable assessment of the patient's competence and level of understanding. The family must be informed of a request by the patient for a DNR order and of the hospital's intention to honor that request. But the family cannot overrule the patient.

The incompetent patient presents a greater challenge. And whatever was true about Grandpa's level of understanding, it was clear to everyone that he was in no position to participate in deliberations about the management of his treatment. The guidelines call for careful assessment of such cases, documentation of the process, and in some instances, prior judicial review. The process differs somewhat according to whether or not the patient is terminally ill. Was this patient terminally ill? I couldn't decide.

He had been stabilized in respect to the immediate trauma of his fall. Without vigorous life-support treatment, providing nutrition, respiration, and response to infection, he would soon die. He could do nothing—literally, chillingly, absolutely nothing—for himself, ever again. His life was over. Yet he was alive and could be kept alive. Somehow, the distinction between patients with terminal illness and other patients seemed far too crude to fit the circumstances.

My thoughts turned to two questions. What is the best outcome we can hope to achieve, and how should it be determined? The guidelines hint at some of the answers, but they leave the hardest questions unsettled, as guidelines and policies always do. How much easier life would be if just once, someone somewhere could write a policy that definitely answered a morally challenging question: Always do this, never do that. The appeal of the idea is easy enough to understand; it is the appeal of simplicity in the face of a complex challenge. But it *never* works. There's always a Grandpa or two, waiting in the wings to thumb their noses at the guidelines by demanding that judgments be made where the guidelines leave off.

The guidelines at Beth Israel reflect this fact; primarily, and quite reasonably, they leave the hardest questions to doctors and family to work out together in the patient's interests. In the Bartling case, no such procedure worked effectively. Sometimes it does.

On Monday, I sit in my office, preparing the first seminar I will give the hospital staff. Will anyone show up, I wonder, already aware of the severe lack of unallocated time in the schedules of hospital workers. And what shall I say to them about ethical issues in health care? Which tip of which iceberg shall I choose?

Some newspaper clippings from last week's Boston Globe *lie on my desk. One headline reads, "New Medical Society life-support policy." The article reports that the Massachusetts Medical Society has decided that it may be acceptable in some cases to withdraw feeding tubes from certain hopelessly ill patients who will die as a result. This new policy has not been announced in any formal way; instead, it has come to light in court testimony on the Brophy case. Brophy is a former fireman who has been comatose for two years. His wife asked that his feeding tube be withdrawn, basing her request on her husband's oft-expressed opposition to being sustained by artificial means. No one is sure what is right to do, so the case is before the courts.*

Another headline, six days later, reads, "Comatose man's

guardian opposes removal of feeding tube." So the dispute goes on.
But it isn't like the Bartling case, for Brophy is long past con-
sciousness. Whatever the outcome of the case, Brophy won't mind.
   I decide to go upstairs to the SICU. The 82-year-old man is gone.
I find the doctor, who tells me that the family decided, after several
visits to the hospital, several conversations with him, and several
conversations among themselves, that a "comfort only" mode of
treatment was appropriate. So a DNR order was written and the
patient was given mild analgesic medication to ease any discom-
fort from the respirator or traction. Two days later he died.

   The decision to forgo life-sustaining treatment must surely be
as hard as any that arises in a hospital or within a family. Principles
to guide such a decision are elusive, because whenever the
question arises, some of our most cherished values are in conflict.
We believe in the value of life, but it is not clear that all life has
value no matter what. We believe that suffering should be reduced, but sometimes that means shortening life. We believe that
patients' wishes should be respected, but that seems not always
best for the patients. We want doctors to be stalwart champions of
life, but we fear their capacity to impose continued life. We want to
be able to say, of a single case, "enough is enough," yet we do not
want to undermine the general respect for life that protects us all.
   The need for clarity about these matters grows steadily as more
and more cases demand such vital decisions. There are several
reasons why. Success at treating various illnesses keeps patients
alive who would otherwise have died; they then can become
potential challenges to medical decision making. New capacities
to sustain life are developed with great frequency; they each have
clear beneficiaries, but they each expand the range of our dilemma. More and more, those in hospitals will be upwards of 85;
many of them will be people of failing health who can be kept alive
despite substantial deterioration. They will be our grandparents,
then our parents, then us.
   In an effort to make a constructive contribution to the discussion of these matters, the federal government conducted an
extensive inquiry into decisions to forgo life-sustaining treatment
(LST). That study was conducted by a short-lived agency named
the President's Commission for the Study of Ethical Problems in

Medicine and Biomedical and Behavioral Research. The commission published eleven reports during its three years of existence; its report on LST, at 554 pages, is by far the largest. It is a sensitive, insightful, humane, and realistic document. But it does not answer the question, "What, in this case, should be done?" Instead, it recognizes that within certain constraints, such decisions must always be made through a process of discussion and reflection involving those persons who are immediately affected by the case.

For that sort of process to be successful, it helps for the various parties to be able to draw on a deep reservoir of prior thought about decisions at the end of life. But too often these questions must be resolved by people thinking about them seriously for the first time.

We gather each day at 11 A.M. in a small conference room on Four North to spend an hour discussing the patients on the unit. The medical students stay put; so does "the Visit," a senior physician who serves as a mentor to the younger physicians. The interns and residents come and go at the whim of their beepers.

Rarely do many minutes go by without that high-pitched staccato intrusion. It is hard to remember that each beep is just the translation of a human call—sometimes of a desperate cry. There's a brief instant of uncertainty and distraction every time. The sound is always the same, so it isn't obvious who is being called. The beepers seem like evil little agents of a conspiracy against rational discourse and unhurried reflection. "Who's got a case?" asks the Visit. Several of the house officers shuffle through their ubiquitous 3 x 5 cards. One of them says, "It's pretty quiet. Mr. L is going home. Nobody's febrile. We had a few admits last night, but nothing special." A few of the patients are discussed very briefly.

A beeper goes off. Two residents, seated beside one another, each reach for their beepers. Everyone else glances, at least briefly, to see who is getting the call. One of the residents pushes the switch on the bleating device; the beeping stops and through the inevitable static a voice instructs, "Call extension 4138." She leaves the room to use the telephone in the hall outside; she may be back in seconds, or not at all.

"How's Mrs. G?" asks the Visit. "Still out of her mind," replies the resident. "We've tapered the steroids and her hematocrit is

still okay, but we don't expect to see improvement in her mental state for several more days."

I'd met Mrs. G a few days earlier. She claimed she was blind, that she'd lost her vision. But she wouldn't open her eyes! Then the head of the medical unit, Dr. L, took her by surprise. "Mrs. G, can you identify that doctor by the door? Do you know him? Have you seen him before?"

She looked, named the doctor, closed her eyes again, and held firm to the claim that she was blind. She also objected that the hospital was trying to starve her, that she'd had no food for days. A nurse whispered to me that Mrs. G had refused to touch breakfast earlier that morning, despite the efforts of the nurse to induce her to eat. Later, the physicians concluded that the most likely explanation of the dementia was a reversible psychosis caused by her medications. The trick would be to reduce her steroids enough to eliminate the mental problems without reducing them too much for her underlying medical problems.

I think, "once again, the Great Pharmacological Balancing Act." The woman comes in sick, and there's no way to tell what dosage will make her better. Put simply, at thirty milligrams, her blood's no good. At forty, her blood's fine, but she's nuts. Is there a place in between, where her blood will still be okay without her being loony? Nobody knows for sure, and the only way to find out is to keep changing the dosages and see what happens. It's all an experiment. She's the subject, and there's no getting out of it.

I wonder how the case will be handled if there is no middle ground, if the only way to keep her in acceptable physical health is going to keep her mind in a mess. I wonder, too, whether some distressed family member might think, "She was sane when she went in, and they've made her crazy. That ought to be worth a million or two." I imagine the headline: "Doctor sued for making patient crazy." I've spent enough time with doctors now that I've started to have malpractice fantasies myself. At the same time, I wonder if these doctors have done all they can to help the patient and family understand how difficult it often is for doctors to figure out what to do. Have they maintained the traditional medical mask of infallible competence? Or they have been open about the limitations of their art?

An intern presents another case, reporting on one of the new admissions. She is 90, and complains of pain in her side. The history shows she's been in before, eleven years ago, for breast cancer. She had a mastectomy and radiation therapy, but rejected advice to start chemotherapy. Now, eleven years later, she's back, coming to the emergency room with a complaint of severe chest pains on awakening. The doctors speak admiringly of her independence of mind, of how she's coming out ahead on her gamble. Once again, their mixed feelings toward powerful drugs are evident.

There's little to be done for her now. She's been ruled out for a myocardial infarction but seems to have metastatic disease. No one speaks in favor of vigorous treatment. "Make her comfortable and send her home," they agree. It is understood that she is likely to be back, when things are worse.

I break my silence on the case. "She's lucid now, seems to have clear opinions about her medical care. The next time she comes in, she might not be. Would it make any sense to find out what her wishes are about medical management while she's able to discuss such things? For instance, how does she feel about DNR orders? She refused chemotherapy; maybe she wouldn't want resuscitation if she came back in bad shape and then arrested. Does anybody know? Will people wait until she arrests to wonder about that?"

I sit back and listen. The residents begin by talking about the diffusion of responsibility. It isn't proper for an intern or a resident to raise such delicate issues with patients; that's the responsibility of the attending physicians, they agree. "The patients don't really view us as their doctors," one of them notes. Yet the attending physicians are themselves reluctant to raise such issues. Quickly, the conversation turns to the difficulty of confronting these matters. One resident turns to the Visit, and asks, "How do you do it? What can you say? I mean, you just can't walk in and say 'Good morning, and by the way, you're in pretty bad shape, you know, and the old ticker could just stop any time now, so what do you want us to do about that? I mean, should we start it up again, or have you had enough?' You can't go in like that. But what can you do?"

For once, the room is silent. Everyone feels the weight of the question. The Visit nods, acknowledging its gravity. Then, gently, he replies.

"To begin with, you can't do it standing up. You must sit down next to the patient. And you have to listen a lot. Sometimes it helps to hold the patient's hand."

He goes on to explain that doctors are afraid of death, of failure, of being blamed. These fears are barriers to discussing death with patients, and consequently with discussing end-stage management. I write in my notes, "If you are dying, remember that your doctor needs all the help you can provide."

The conversation continues for fifteen minutes. I listen with admiration; these are caring, sensitive, intelligent people, pursuing an issue that causes them pain, but that they cannot avoid. I am content to let the discussion run its course.

It is noon; and the clock rules. The conference ends and we disperse. In the hall, I catch up to one of the residents and ask him how often he has participated in such discussions in his training. He stops and seems to turn inward for an instant. Then he replies: "Well, of course, I have to deal with those problems when they come up. And it isn't easy, but I do the best I can. As far as having the chance to talk about it like that, well, I've been here for three years, and it's never happened before."

Some patients are so ill that regardless of their own previously expressed views toward the prolongation of life, the physicians treating them believe, or are at least tempted to believe, that the allocation of human and economic resources to that treatment cannot be justified. This is an extremely discomforting attitude for health care providers to have; the culture of medicine has long held that the physician's obligation is to serve the interest of the patient, whatever the cost, and that questions about the allocation of resources can comfortably be set aside for others to address (or for physicians to consider in their capacity as citizens, apart from the context of the treatment of particular patients). But medicine's increasing capacity to sustain life in the face of dismal prognoses makes the question of resource allocation harder and harder to avoid in clinical settings.

The issue arises most clearly in intensive care units, which provide the hospital's costliest context of care. (In one hospital, in which the ICUs include less than 9% of the beds and provide less than 8% of the patient-bed-days—a patient in a bed for a day, over 20% of the total hospital budget and of nursing staff time are absorbed by the ICUs.) This is no surprise; that's where the sickest people are, which is why the care, and the costs, are intensive. Despite a national surplus in total hospital beds available, ICU resources are sometimes in great demand. Yet, because they are the most costly resources, they are the hardest to expand.

The problem is especially acute in urban, public hospitals, where occupancies are increasing in part because of more numerous transfers of the uninsured to such hospitals. There have even been confirmed instances of such patients who, having failed the wallet biopsy in the emergency room of a private hospital, were transferred to public hospitals while still in mortal danger. As public hospitals increasingly become a sort of *de facto* national health insurance system, compensating for our collective negligence at the national level, the financial pressures on them increase, and their ability to enlarge their capacity diminishes.

Serious perils attend this situation. In one case, a hospital admitted the victim of a terrible automobile accident, despite the fact that the ICU was already filled beyond its normal capacity. The patient did badly and a lawsuit resulted. In the trial, knowing that the hospital had provided less intensive ICU care than the normal census would have allowed, the jury awarded the plaintiff twelve million dollars. That seems to provide a strong argument for locking the doors when the ICU is full, and perhaps posting a "no vacancy" sign in front of the emergency room. But some doctors are beginning to consider a different way of addressing the problem.

The speaker at the anesthesia department's lecture on ethics and intensive care is the director of an ICU at one of the other Harvard teaching hospitals. He describes the current difficulties as he experiences them, emphasizing the apparent irrationality of turning away a patient with good prospects for recovery just because an ICU is already filled, when some of those filling it are nearly hopeless cases. He proposes that the custom of respecting seniority in the ICU—the "first come, first served, and once served entitled to remain" principle of access—be replaced by the adoption of an "Intensive Care Entitlement Index," according to which each patient's prospects for recovery would be assessed, perhaps daily, with ICU space to be made available according to the patient's index. Too low an index could result in refusal of access; it could also result in removal from the unit in favor of a newcomer with a higher index. It is not obvious that any such index can be coherently determined, but the speaker suggests various formulations of how it might be calculated.

A questioner challenges the necessity for such a radical departure. The speaker replies by describing one of the experiences that prompted him to rethink how access to the unit is allocated. A 21-year-old male, struck by lightning, had excellent prospects for recovery, but was turned away because the ICU was full. At the time, there were five patients in the unit who had no significant prospect of recovery. They were kept alive because it was possible, not because it made sense. And the prospective patient had no recourse in competition with those who outranked him simply by getting into the unit sooner. (Perhaps the young man survived the delay and was treated successfully elsewhere; we are not told.)

The debate continues, with several physicians either challenging the possibility of devising any such index or raising alarms about its possible misuse. The scheme strikes me as preposterous; I have visions of people being moved in and out of ICUs the way teams move in and out of first place. But is that any less preposterous than what the present situation allows?

A doctor comments who is troubled by the problem and by this proposed solution. These matters cannot be resolved by doctors, but must merely be raised by them, he argues. "We have to project these questions into the public arena, so that a public negotiation will ensue," he concludes. The visiting speaker agrees. And then he goes back to his ICU to treat the patients already there and to worry about those who may be on the way.

Many grievously ill patients are saved by the treatment they receive in ICUs. Some return to complete health. Even with the best of care, however, some patients die. Dealing with their deaths and with their families is a painful part of the reality in the hospital.

It can be especially difficult when the death is clouded by the use of life-support systems which must be deliberately withdrawn.

I meet with a nursing administrator, Ms. F, who expresses her concern that as economic and legal issues increasingly dominate the agendas of hospital administrators, they will become increasingly removed from patients, and therefore from "what the real issues are."

She tells me of a case about a year ago. A young woman, grievously injured, was in critical condition, on life-support equipment. During the period of uncertainty, Ms. F had sat with members of the family, helping them deal with their ordeal. When the young woman was declared brain dead, it was time to turn off the life-support system; she satisfied the legal definition of death, and was thus no longer a patient. But the family found this impossible to accept.

The health care team then met with the family. Including a boyfriend, a minister, and some aunts and uncles, they numbered about a dozen. They were joined by seven or eight people from the hospital who had cared for the woman, including three physicians and two nurses. During the meeting, which lasted about an hour, the hospital staff explained the reality to the family. The family turned its attention to the need to pick a time for the cessation of life support, and asked for twelve more hours to allow additional visits. The staff agreed. The minister spoke of the woman's life and of her children, as the grieving process began. The woman was to be moved to an isolated unit, with no restrictions placed on the family's final visits. Disconnection was scheduled for the following morning. The staff withdrew to allow the family to meet in private. The staff then returned, and the woman's father sadly told the surgeon, "You have our permission." The surgeon left in silence.

There are tears in Ms. F's eyes as she tells the story, and in mine as I hear it. She is still moved, a year later, by the family's pain and also by the response of a community of caregivers to that pain. It is the kind of response she and her staff want to be able always to provide, but doing so gets harder and harder. The story, which provides a model of sensitivity and humane concern, depends on a contribution of uncompensated time by many busy people from the hospital. How can such behavior be sustained, we both wonder, as economic pressures increase the demand for greater efficiency in hospital care?

Ms. F continues. "Often the physicians just can't see, once they've made their clinical decision—even if that takes five days—why there is then any delay." She illustrates the problem with a second case. A young man, injured in a two-story fall, came out of surgery brain dead. The surgeons told his sister, who was next of kin, that he would not recover. She became hysterical and incoherent. But she returned the next day —assuming she would be a part of the decision to disconnect the life-support system—saying "I think I can deal with it now." By then the body was already in the morgue.

"How could we handle that case so badly," Ms. F asks, "after we handled the first one so well? There is the clinical, technical piece, and then there is all the rest—which is so important!" But we both know that it will be a fierce battle to protect the time and resources needed to attend to the rest, and that the nursing staff will be in the vanguard of that battle.

As contemporary health care confronts the increasingly difficult issues that arise at the end of life, there are many situations in which we are inclined or even feel compelled to ask where the line should be drawn—between respecting a patient's autonomy and serving that patient's interest, between meeting all identifiable medical needs and breaking the bank, between saving a life and prolonging a dying. All these issues require the making of difficult judgments in the absence of definitive rules or guidelines. The general cultural context—a complex of evolving societal values, conventions of medical and nursing practice, laws and legal precedents—and the particulars of the situation at hand, interact to determine a band of uncertainty within which the judgment must be made. No algorithm eliminates this necessity, because none is adequately sensitive to the variability of the human realities at the end of life. In these situations it is never clear where to draw the line. And sometimes it is best not even to ask.

As we walk around the unit, the resident gives me a quick summary of each case. In one room, a gaunt, grey woman in her late sixties sits gasping in her oxygen tent, her barely audible cry of "Help, help, help" repeated over and over. The resident says "That's Mrs. B," but ignores her supplications.

"Can't you do something for her?" I ask.

He leads me out of the room, explaining, "Heavy smoker. End stage emphysema. Nothing anyone can do. She says that all the time. But she's just suffocating to death, and it won't be very long. Terrible way to go."

"What about comfort? Narcotics?"

"I'm going to ask the attending later. Maybe we can increase it."

The next day, Friday, I find her sleeping, and learn that a morphine drip has been added to her IV. Her breathing is extremely shallow. On Monday, the bed is empty. "Mrs. B?" I ask.

"Died," the nurse replies. "Finally." The bed is empty, but the image remains strong of Mrs. B, hopelessly rasping, futilely imploring, helplessly sinking.

Later, I see the resident, and mention that Mrs. B seemed not to be suffering the last time I saw her. "Yes," he said, "we decided to increase the morphine."

"Doesn't that suppress the respiration," I ask.

"Sure, somewhat."

"Enough, maybe, to hasten the death considerably?"

"Hard to say," he replies. "Hard to say."

The next week, walking into the garage, I see one of the nurses leaving in her car. She is in her twenties, very bright, youthful, attractive. She is smoking. I stand there, watching as she drives past me, changing before my eyes into Mrs. B.

8
. . .

MARKETING
HEALTH
CARE

*T*he Executive Committee of the Board of Trustees meets in a comfortable conference room adjacent to the president's office. No major or controversial decisions are pending; the meeting is largely informational. Dr. Rabkin talks about Beth Israel's relationship with other hospitals in the area and with the Harvard Community Health Plan—a local health maintenance organization only very loosely connected with Harvard. Increasingly, he emphasizes, control of health care institutions is shifting to individuals as employers offer their workers a more diverse array of health care plans of varying costs and qualities. He reports on the progress of search committees seeking to fill vacant positions in two departments, on sabbatical plans for a few staff physicians, and on the status of discussions about the possible medical uses of a vacant building in the vicinity. Various financial and business officers then each offer reports in turn.

There is some good news; the current phase of construction will be completed below budget by several million dollars, which can be applied to the next phase. The new dialysis unit has just opened, and the hospital's request for an increased payment rate for dialysis treatment has been partially granted (the costs of dialysis are paid by the federal government according to an approved schedule of charges). That request had been pending since its

126

submission a year and a half earlier; it is welcome news that the increased rate has been approved retroactively, even though the increase is somewhat less than requested. Dialysis patients at Beth Israel are older and sicker than dialysis patients at most other hospitals, so it is more costly to treat them. This point has finally been accepted as a basis for changing the payment schedule.

Health care, we are told, is marching forward faster each week into the competitive arena of seeking business. An assistant for planning and marketing explains that hospitals have historically functioned largely on the basis of the needs and wants of health care providers and the hospital as an institution. Now this pattern is under heavy pressure to change. For example, it is becoming necessary to have office hours in pediatrics in the evening to accommodate the needs of working mothers; hospitals resistant to the change will be left behind as medical care adapts to the increasingly competitive market. (Beth Israel does not have a pediatrics unit, however.)

This hospital, we learn, shows signs of doing well overall. The average length of stay is low and occupancy is increasing at a time when many other hospitals have a decreasing occupancy rate. This is encouraging in regard to prospects for future pricing—an advantage in the competitive arena. "We're looking like winners," notes one of the administrators. There is talk of a "competitor scan" and of the need to "define the product" clearly.

Dr. Rabkin emphasizes the importance of maintaining a cooperative attitude regarding the several neighboring hospitals in the Longwood medical complex. Possibly the vacant building next door, formerly the Massachusetts College of Art, can be acquired for some common purpose, for example, rather than being the object of competition among the various nearby hospitals. Perhaps these hospitals can work together to increase the role they play regionally, rather than competing with one another for patients.

A trustee is struck by the tone of the discussion. (I have been wondering whether it would sound very different at a meeting of Sears, Roebuck or Procter & Gamble.) She suggests that this competitive situation is simply contrary to the requirements of good health care, which is dependent on structures of cooperation and sensitivity to patients' needs. Yet she recognizes the reality of the financial pressures on the hospital.

Here is a hospital that should be at the pinnacle of the health care system. It is a teaching unit of a medical school as prestigious as any, it has a reputation for extraordinarily good patient care, its nursing staff and program are nationally hailed as exemplary, it has strong financial support from a generous and affluent constituency, it is untainted by the profit motive, and here we sit talking about competitor scans, product definition, market position, and other aspects of the fight for financial survival. Can it be that even this hospital will one day be hustling for business? Will there be a sales force, advertising, promotional incentives, discount coupons?

The economic pressures on health care providers and institutions are rapidly growing more pervasive and visible. Many factors, apart from inflation, contribute to this increasing presence of economic concerns in discussions about medical care. Some of these factors are traditional marketplace phenomena—for example, nurses, tired of being an underpaid profession, have sought wage increases that greatly exceed the rate of inflation. And those increases must be provided, now that the profession of nursing is no longer artificially supported by pervasive discrimination against women in other professions. Indeed, the national shortage of nurses is critical in some locations, and nurses' salaries at some hospitals have increased by over 30% in the past three years as a result. The price of liability protection has soared as a result of the increasing frequency of multimillion dollar judgments against health care providers in malpractice cases; the cost of these judgments and premiums significantly raises the price of health care services. So do the costs of medical tests that are done not because they are medically advised but because they strengthen the evidence—just in case it is needed—that the physician has been absolutely thorough.

Medical progress itself sometimes contributes to the problem. Although many medical advances make it less costly to treat a particular class of patients, other advances in health care increase the powers of medical intervention in ways that also increase costs. An example of the former is the development of new immunosuppressive drugs, which greatly increase the success rate for organ transplantation. Since it is far less costly to maintain a patient after a successful kidney transplant than to maintain that patient on renal dialysis, the availability of such drugs is an advance that saves money.

Other advances, however, require immense expenditures. We need not look to exotic experimental devices like the artificial heart to find this effect. The CAT scan equipment that became widely available in the 1970s required an investment of millions on the part of each hospital or medical unit that acquired it. Now magnetic resonance imaging devices offer a superior technology—sharper images without radiation risks, but this new equipment is even more costly.

Many couples who earlier would have had to live with their infertility, either remaining childless or else adopting children, now are patients at *in vitro* fertilization programs sometimes costing tens of thousands of dollars. Victims who would have died at the scene of an accident or assault a few years ago are now rushed by helicopter to shock trauma units where their lives may be saved by extremely intensive care that is immensely expensive. New drugs, developed only after long and costly research programs, require long and costly testing before they are approved for use as safe and effective; when they are finally on the market, they are priced to include the costs of research and testing, in addition to those of production, marketing, liability protection, and profit margin.

So the costs of medical care climb higher and higher, at a time of increasing pressure from various sources to contain them. That pressure is not a reaction only to higher health care costs. It is that in part, but it is also due in part to such factors as concern with the weakness of the national economy that is reflected in an enormous federal deficit and our unfavorable international trading position.

To compete successfully with foreign manufacturers who have both highly efficient production technology and a very inexpensive labor force, American manufacturers must lower their production costs in every possible way. A major ingredient in the per-unit production costs of American manufactured goods—especially heavy goods such as automobiles and appliances—is the cost of health care insurance for employees. So employers want to contain or even reduce the cost of health care plans. The only ways to do that are to reduce coverage, increase efficiency, and reduce or externalize the actual costs of medical care. All these methods are being tried, but there is understandably great resistance to reductions in coverage, especially as the costs of care are increasing. And only a limited amount can be achieved through increased efficiency. So limiting the costs of health care becomes a major focus. This concern has become so great that several chief executive officers of major industrial corporations have recently called for an increased federal role in meeting health care needs. Since the absence of any national health insurance plan in the United States places us at a distinct disadvantage in competition with industries in other countries that need not incorporate health care costs in their pricing structures, the leaders of American business may become the force for social change that the advocates for disadvantaged populations have been unable to become.

At the federal level, there has long been some concern for that 15% of the American population who lack adequate access to decent medical care because of their poverty, but there was even greater concern, at least within the Reagan administration, to reduce total federal expenditures for social programs. Thus President Reagan, in his budget request for fiscal year 1987, tried to cut seventy billion dollars from federal outlays for health care.

The pressures that increase medical costs and the pressures to reduce them are thus on a collision course, with hospitals uncomfortably in the middle—most with decreasing occupancy rates that mean lower income in the face of rising costs. No wonder they are starting to think of the world of prospective patients as the marketplace; no wonder they are becoming more aggressively competitive with one another. No wonder that advertising has become a basic part of the marketing program at many hospitals around the country.

"WE CAN'T WAIT TO GET YOU INTO OUR NEW OPERAT-ING ROOM" reads the headline of an advertisement by Virginia Beach General Hospital. The smaller print reveals that the hospital plans an open house to show the public its new surgical suites. I see a reprint of the ad in the latest issue of Healthcare Advertis-

ing Review, *which describes the ad as "calculated shock." The
review comments admiringly that "The headline was, obviously,
deliberately intended to shock people into a major bit of reading,
even if it had to turn a few people off to do it. How well did it work?
Over 800 people attended VBGH's open house . . . and we really
like the quality of the copy."*

*Another headline catches my eye. "ATTENTION MEDICARE
PATIENTS," says the First Stop Medical Clinic of Racine, Wis-
consin, and, below, "This coupon is worth $100 toward a complete
medical examination." A discount coupon! The review's comment
has a headline of its own, "HARD SELL . . . SELLS." Indeed it
does; I read that "Ten to twenty new patients a day come walking
into First Stop's 13 clinics, each holding a $100 coupon . . . and
each one a potential avenue to hundreds or thousands of dollars in
Medicare and/or other third-party payments. A&P has been using
this format to sell soup and soap and soda pop for years; now First
Stop brings the 'cents-off' coupon to patients in their Golden
Years."*

*Finally I get to the front of the magazine; I see that I can
subscribe for $185 a year. The copy tells me why I should: "Bring
in the patients; bring in the profits! That's the undisguised goal of
some of the finest advertising and promotion being done in
America today." But I decide to do without its systematic collection of the best; I'll settle for what I come across on my own.*

The rush toward aggressive health care marketing will surely
continue, as the old restraints against advertising by professionals
crumble away—much to the sadness of many doctors, lawyers,
and hospital administrators whose sense of the dignity of their
professions is assaulted by such developments. But their resistance is to little avail.

In *Bates v. State Bar of Arizona* (433 U.S. 350, 1977), the
Supreme Court extended first amendment protection to advertising by attorneys. The Bar Association of Arizona had argued
against that extension, claiming that advertising by attorneys
would have adverse effects on professionalism, would be inherently misleading, would promote groundless litigation, would
increase costs, would lead to undesirable packaging of fixed price
services, and would lead to extreme problems of enforcement. The

Court found these claims to be without substance. But it held, importantly, that it is the duty of the Bar Association to ensure full disclosure in all legal advertising and to promote consumer education with respect to legal services. Further, the Court said that

> Because of the complexity of legal services and the lack of public sophistication, higher standards of truth than those applicable to other forms of commercial speech might apply. In some situations, supplements to advertisements, such as of warnings or disclaimers, may be required to prevent deception. Finally, claims concerning the quality of legal services which cannot be verified may be prohibited as misleading.

More recently, the Virginia Code of Professional Responsibility was modified to allow attorneys to advertise without restriction, so long as the advertisements contain "no false, fraudulent, or deceptive claim or statement." So an attorney in Virginia may advertise that she wins 97% of her cases, or that her settlements are on the average 17% larger than the norm for attorneys in the region with comparable types of practice, so long as such claims are not false, fraudulent, or deceptive.

Legal advertising is clearly on the rise and is a part of the reality of professional competition. But health care advertising, a bit slower out of the starting gate, has now taken the lead in the area of professional services. Is this a problem? Need anything be done about it? What does it portend for hospitals like Boston's Beth Israel? We can approach these questions by considering what might be said in such advertisements, what it may be taken to mean, what dangers can arise, and what measures might be appropriate against such dangers.

More may well be necessary than reliance on the integrity of professionals, hospitals, the advertising agencies, and the media. We hear affirmations of integrity in all those quarters, but complacent reliance on them is unwise. Many—perhaps the vast majority—of profit-oriented executives are people of integrity who want to make money in a way that is honest and serves the public interest. Many copywriters will only write advertisements that are in good taste, and many newspapers will refuse to run ads that are deficient in any of a long list of respects. Most people are decent folks in most respects most of the time.

Still, some behavior occurs nearer the edges of the statistical distribution. So we have laws against arson, looting, and assault, without suggesting that they are necessary to keep most people from behaving badly. And we have regulations to protect us against various kinds of malfeasance, not because we think they are likely, but because we know they are possible. We construct protections against damaging and deviant behavior in various domains of activity, without indictment of those domains as a whole. Even if most advertising is admirable—a claim I would not want to have to defend—it is still wise to consider the possible pitfalls associated with unrestrained, irresponsible professional advertising. This, I believe, is the perspective reflected in the Court's imposition of regulatory responsibilities on the Arizona Bar Association.

Physicians do not yet typically advertise as independent practitioners, but many hospitals have become prominent advertisers of their services and facilities as the competition for patients increases.

At a meeting of the administrative staff, the discussion focuses on the impact of the hospital's financial dependence on the DRGs in which the patients are classified. All Medicare payments are based on DRG assignments, and 40% of this hospital's cash flow is from Medicare. So a great amount depends on the particulars of the processes of DRG classification. For example, the payment for a patient can vary by as much as $2000 depending on the presence or absence of anemia in the diagnosis.

There is obviously an incentive for the hospital to find, for each patient, the diagnosis that will yield the highest rate of reimbursement. Much of this process is now computerized; the diagnostic information is the input and the appropriate DRG classification is the output. The software presumably makes the optimal classification consistent with the medical facts.

One physician advises, "It is important always to ask, 'Can the DRG be upgraded truthfully on the basis of the laboratory values?'" He is not suggesting misrepresentation in any way, but is adding a new responsibility to the physician's traditional concerns—the responsibility to respect the hospital's financial interests by making diagnostic choices, consistent with the medical facts, that are sensitive to the financial consequences of subtle diagnostic differences. If a patient's blood count is at the margin of what can reasonably be called anemia, there is a positive incentive for adding that to the diagnosis on the record.

There is a corresponding incentive on the part of the payer to be vigilant in scrutiny of the legitimacy of the diagnoses, so that no "DRG gaming" occurs to their disadvantage—especially as the particulars of a diagnosis are often probabilistic judgments made in a context of considerable uncertainty. This vigilance, a hospital administrator points out, may soon be reflected in a decision by the Health Care Financing Administration to examine the DRG software used by hospitals. Dr. Rabkin notes ironically, "Soon the world will consist entirely of auditors; no one will be doing anything."

The discussion turns to the importance of marketing the hospital's services to the well-to-do. I learn that the hospital has a close association with Clinica Boston in Madrid, which is a source of wealthy patients primarily from the Jewish community in Spain. Such patients deposit funds in advance sufficient to cover the estimated costs of their hospitalizations. The notion is raised of marketing the hospital's services to wealthy Jewish populations in other European countries. An influential state legislator, a member of the Massachusetts State International Coordinating Council, is at work on increasing European trade for Massachusetts, and sees Boston's hospitals as playing an important role.

Again, the question is raised of defining the product, only this time it is raised by a physician. "Is it medical scholarship, patient care, the number of admits, or the bottom line? What is the mix?" There is more discussion of the climate of competition, not only for individual patients but for association with the increasingly powerful health maintenance organizations that represent large blocks of patients. One speaker invokes the metaphor of circling the wagons. Dr. Rabkin reiterates the value of attracting more business from outside the immediate region, rather than compet-

ing with other Boston area hospitals for local business. "Two dogs can't get fat eating each other's fleas," he concludes.

To facilitate speculation about where all this might lead, consider two hypothetical advertisements I wrote as heuristic examples, with no suggestion that any specific advertiser might use them. Imagine that they appear in your local newspaper.

The first one reads as follows.

An important notice from the Wholesome Hospital Corporation

SAFE!   EFFECTIVE!   SIMPLE!

Tired of tiny tots? Fed up with inconvenience and uncertainty?

Sign up now for our special

WEEKEND ESCAPE

All at one low package price, we will tie your tubes, and provide all related services including a deluxe room with color TV and telephone, and all meals. Transportation optional. Then, just three weeks later, at no extra charge . . .

Enjoy your new freedom at the nearby Eros Lodge Hotel with the guest of your choice, for two glorious days and one night, including continental breakfast for two and a welcoming bottle of champagne!

DON'T PROCRASTINATE; DON'T PROCREATE
Call our toll-free number now; major credit cards accepted.
800-010-0000
(Men! Ask about our Vasectomy Value Vacation.)

Read these testimonials from satisfied clients!
Mrs. H.G. It was the best anniversary present Leo ever gave me.
Ms. W.N. I don't know why I waited so long. Your weekend special changed my life!
Mrs. R.V. I recommend you to all my friends. And to think the health insurance paid for it all! It's the best value around.
When it comes to your health, the Wholesome Hospital Corporation is always a step ahead!

I wrote that just to get into a copywriting frame of mind, and to get a sense of what might happen if hospital advertising became aggressive and unrestrained, even by canons of good taste. Of course no hospital would actually place such an ad. But it can be useful to have an example of what is clearly beyond the limits of appropriateness.

The second example is less obviously unrealistic.

An Important Message
to
HEART PATIENTS
from the
Wholesome Hospital Corporation

Last year hundreds of patients had elective heart surgery at Wholesome Hospital. Nearly all of them returned to good health. In fact, the mortality rate was just 2%. Hundreds of patients had heart surgery at Urban Central Hospital, too. But the mortality rate there was *300% higher!* In that teaching hospital, lots of young doctors and medical students are in training. At the Wholesome Hospital, only fully qualified surgeons are permitted to perform surgery.
The choice is yours.
When the time comes to schedule your bypass surgery, call us directly, or tell your doctor that you prefer Wholesome Hospital, the one with the high rate of success. And remember: When it comes to your health, the Wholesome Hospital Corporation is always a step ahead.

(Medicaid patients not accepted.)

This advertisement, too, would distress me if it were actually placed by a hospital, despite the fact that (by hypothesis) there is no false claim within it. But it is not enough simply to judge an advertisement objectionable; the point is to clarify precisely just what about it is distressing. Knowing that may help us understand what limits, if any, to place on a hospital's freedom to advertise, or what limits to accept voluntarily about what one will or will not do in response to competition—and this is an issue that Boston's Beth Israel will surely have to confront as it seeks to draw a delicate line between meeting the realities of its economic environment and sacrificing its traditions as a provider of care.

To understand better how to get some endeavor right, it generally makes sense to look at examples of its going wrong, and to clarify what is wrong about them. One way to understand the ingredients of good medical practice is to examine specific instances of bad medical practice, identifying and analyzing their deficiencies; the same approach can shed light on advertising practices in health care.

The advertisement for heart surgery is misleading in various ways, without resorting to falsehood. Studies of coronary arterial bypass surgery do indicate a range of mortality rates roughly from 2% to 6%. So Wholesome Hospital's (WH) mortality rate could well be 2%, while the rate at Urban Central (UC) could be 6%. But note that the rate given for WH is for elective surgery, while that given for UC is for all heart surgery. That difference alone could account for a difference in mortality rates.

The suggestion in the ad is that the difference in rates reflects a difference in quality of care, but it may reflect nothing more than a difference in the patient populations. This possibility is reinforced by the fact that WH declines to serve Medicaid patients, who are therefore likely to be a part of the UC population, and are also likely to be a population with poorer health and lower prospects of recovery. One very effective way of maintaining a high success rate is to refuse to take the very difficult cases, sending them instead to public hospitals which do not have the same luxury of turning them away.

Note also the suggestion implicit in the comment about staff responsibilities. True, UC—like Beth Israel—is a teaching hospital. It is also true that at WH only fully qualified surgeons are permitted to perform surgery. One is invited to infer that at UC surgery is performed by the unqualified. But that is likely untrue. It may be that surgery is performed in part by surgeons in training under the supervision of more senior physicians, but it is not obvious either that they are therefore unqualified, or even that the standard of care is in any way lower than at WH. Indeed, it may even be that the combination of distinguished clinical faculty and surgeons-in-training, working under close scrutiny at UC, provides a higher level of skill overall than do the practitioners at WH.

Finally, note how the figures are presented. A mortality rate of 6% is obviously higher than one of 2%, although it is still fairly low. But the figure of 6% does not appear in the advertisement. Instead, we are told that the UC rate is "300% higher"—a dramatic difference indeed! The same statistics could be presented differently, of course. It could have been claimed that the success rate at UC is only 94%, while at WH it is 98%. That may be a significant difference, but putting the figures that way makes it plain that both hospitals have low mortality rates, and similar success rates. The advertisement is written to take advantage of the fact that statistical literacy is extremely rare and that these two different ways of representing the same data will have very different impacts on typical readers. Thus, the reference to WH as "The one with the high rate of success" reinforces the misimpression that UC has a low rate.

It is time to give my first seminar in the hospital. I gather my notes and papers, and head for the seminar room. About forty people are there, a mix of doctors, nurses, students, health administrators, and miscellaneous tourists. I put them to work on an exercise designed to reveal how tenuous and unreliable our instincts about statistical matters tend to be. I ask them each to answer two questions on a handout sheet, and promise to report on their responses the next week. They have plenty of time; the sheet is passed out at the beginning of the seminar and won't be collected until the end.

Here is a slightly revised version of that handout.

Assume that the following information is true.

A new disease affecting people who read books about health care has recently been identified. It occurs in .1% of the population at risk. The symptoms are nasty, but the disease is not fatal. If it is left untreated, the victim has chills and fever for several weeks and suffers from moderate intermittent nausea and palsy. The symptoms then diminish and disappear. A new treatment eliminates these symptoms entirely, but it only works if administered prior to the onset of symptoms. That treatment involves no significant risk, and nearly always works. But it is costly, involves taking daily doses of a foul medicine, and, worse, requires total abstention from ice cream for eight weeks.

A new test has been developed to identify victims of the disease presymptomatically. Its specificity and sensitivity are each 98%; that is, it identifies 98% of those who have the disease with a positive test result, and it identifies 98% of those who do not have the disease with a negative test result.

The public health service has screened 100,000 potential victims of the disease with this test, in order to identify those who should be offered the treatment.

I regret to inform you that your test was positive. Please answer these two questions.

    1. How likely do you think it is that you have the disease? Probability: (check one) 95% + _____, 85–94% _____, 74–84% _____, 65–74% _____, 55–64% _____, 45–54% _____, 35–44% _____, 25–34% _____, 15–24% _____, 5–14% _____, 1–5% _____, 0% _____.
    2. Do you want the treatment?

Take a few moments now to answer these questions for yourself. You need not calculate the answer to (1); just estimate what seems most reasonable. And you need not justify your answer to (2). I'll tell you in a few pages how the Beth Israel group answered, and how to think correctly about these questions. In the meantime, return to the advertisement by Wholesome Hospital.

This advertisement is misleading, so it would clearly be prohibited by any standard that effectively prohibits misleading claims. Would it be barred by regulations like that governing legal advertising in Virginia, which merely forbids "false, fraudulent, or deceptive" claims or statements? The advertisement contains no false claims, so the question turns on whether it is fraudulent or deceptive overall. That will depend upon how strictly the notions of fraud, deceit, and the misleading are interpreted, as well as on the effectiveness of monitoring and enforcement. A very strict interpretation might be hard to sustain, given the abundance of misleading advertising that surrounds us.

The advertisement is hypothetical, but the competitive phenomenon it reflects is not. The incursion of private for-profit hospitals into the market in competition with public hospitals has already resulted in fierce competition, with private hospitals sometimes skimming off the more profitable cases, leaving the public hospitals with a greater proportion of patients whose prospects of recovery are least or who cannot cover the costs of their care. The impact of the Wholesome Hospitals thus functions, at least in part, contrary to the public interest, though perhaps profitably for their stockholders.

Although the development of the for-profit hospital sector has not yet had a major impact in Massachusetts, it is very much a part of the health care scene in many other regions, and it may one day become significant in Beth Israel's market. Even without it, some hospitals in the Boston area already advertise for patients. Such competition has prompted very aggressive advertising campaigns in some regions.

An article in *The Miami News* (April 9, 1984) under the headline "Hospitals vie for patients with Madison Avenue flair," reported that ten major hospitals in the area were spending $100,000 to $400,000 on annual advertising budgets—roughly twenty times what was spent just three years earlier. Most of the advertising is positive in tone, simply emphasizing the virtues of what the hospitals provide. But the article quotes Ken Magee of the Florida Hospital Association as saying, "We really are in a competitive marketplace right now. . . . I think you will start to see some cutthroat competition, the kind that goes on in almost every marketplace."

Back in my office, I tally the responses to my two questions about the hypothetical disease. Doctors and nurses, about two-thirds of the audience, were present in equal numbers—fourteen of each. Most of the doctors (over 60% of them) indicate that the likelihood of their having the disease, given the positive test result, is at least 95%. All but one of them judges the likelihood to be at least 85%. That one deviant respondent thinks it no more than 5%!

The nurses' views are more dispersed. Only 57% of them say the odds are at least 85%, and there are two maverick nurses who vote with the one dissenting doctor. The leftovers—neither doctor nor nurse—react somewhat differently. One-third of them (probably not a statistically significant number) say that the odds are not over 5%.

I notice a high correlation between answers to the first question and answers to the second one. The more likely a person thinks it is that he or she has the disease, the more likely it is that he or she has chosen the treatment. But there are exceptions; some of those who think the probability high nonetheless decline the treatment.

What the probability actually is can be calculated; it is a matter of demonstrable fact, not open to dispute. How a person responds to a treatment option is a different sort of matter; it just isn't possible to get the second question demonstrably wrong. It's one of those value questions about a medical decision that is based on the relevant facts, but not derivable from them.

Here, the factual and value aspects are separated into questions 1 and 2. No one seems confused about the difference between them; no one suggests that if the probability is high, it is a fact that treatment should be accepted. In the real world of medical care, facts and values swirl around together. It is easy to get them confused, and judgments about values are often disguised as statements of fact.

These figures do not surprise me. Sound statistical judgment is exceedingly rare, and I have used the exercise to make that point vividly to the Beth Israel staff. At the same time, I realize that it would have been comforting to find that these health care professionals are an exception.

I've promised to tell them next week about the exercise. It would be a great embarrassment to get it wrong myself when I tell them that most of them have gotten it wrong. So I decide to run through the figures one more time.

The incidence of the disease is one-tenth of 1% of the population. So of the 100,000 people who have been screened, 100 (approximately) have the disease. The test identifies 98% of the disease victims with a positive test result, so it will produce 98 positives—true positives—from those 100 people. The remaining 99,900 screened people do not have the disease, and the test will show that fact by providing most of them (98% of them) with a negative test result—a true negative.

But the test isn't quite perfect; it will fail to identify 2% of those who are disease free as being disease free. It will give them a positive result—a false positive—even though they do not have the disease. Since there are 99,900 without the disease, that 2% rate of false positives will yield 1,998 more positive results, all of them false. The total number of positives based on the screening of 100,000 people will therefore be 1,998 plus 98, or 2096. But of these 2096 positives, only 98—4.7% of them—will be true positives! So on the basis of the data provided in the statement of the problem, the likelihood of a person in the population at risk actually having the disease, given a positive screening test result, is less than 5%.

"Bravo!" for the dissenting doctor and the two maverick nurses. I'll go through the calculations at the next seminar, emphasizing that the point is not to embarrass anyone, but to underscore how pervasively devoid of even elementary statistical sense most people, including health care professionals, are. Medical education does not produce statistical literacy, even though medical decisions are largely based on statistics.

Consider now an actual advertisement placed by a medical center in *The Miami Herald* (April 10, 1984). The ad invites readers to free cancer screenings, claiming that "Last year we identified 427 suspected cancers after screening more than 2000 people." How are we to interpret such a claim? Grant that it is good for free screenings to be available and for people to take advantage of them. Consider what this advertisement says. The initial impact is that over 20% of those screened have suspected cancer—if we assume that "more than 2000" stands for some number very close to 2000. If the actual number of people screened is much larger, the inference to a percentage will be proportionally erroneous. But even if the actual number is 2001, the impression given may be very misleading. For the advertisement says nothing about the screening technique used, so we have no information about its accuracy.

Assume that the actual rate of disease in the screened population is 3%. Then, of the 2000 subjects, 60 will have some relevant form of cancer. Assume further that the screening technique has a 98% sensitivity—that is, that it accurately identifies 98% of those who are afflicted. The process will then have identified 59 of the 60 cancer victims with positive test results. Add just one further assumption—that the screening technique has achieved its high sensitivity at the cost of achieving only a modest selectivity; it correctly yields a negative test result for 81% of those who are disease free. Then, of the 1940 healthy individuals screened, 19%, or 368, will also have positive test results, although they will be false positives. The total number of positive tests will thus be 427, as advertised. But of those 427 who are identified as suspected cancers, only 59—14%—will actually be ill. The other 86% of those who tested positive—368 people—will presumably go through some considerable terror before subsequently being confirmed as false positives, and perhaps some of them will even be subjected to costly or harmful treatments for a disease they do not have.

It may well be worth subjecting them to that distress and risk in order to identify and help the 59 people who are diseased. Still, in deciding whether to present oneself for such screening, one might reasonably want to know about the incidence of the disease, the accuracy of the screening technique, and the availability of reliable methods of confirmation of initial test results. Perhaps the actual technique that was used is vastly better than what I have assumed here for illustrative analysis. But there is no way to know that from the advertisement.

The medical center placing the advertisement had dual motivation. It wants to contribute to good health by identifying people who need treatment. But it also very much wants to be the provider of that and other treatments. So the screening program also serves as a way of building connections with the community and of increasing the center's visibility. Thus, the advertisement also says, "Discover the New North Shore Medical Center." That is an entirely reasonable objective, but it conflicts with the disclosure of information about the screening program that might decrease the reader's inclination to go to the center to participate in the program.

I don't condemn this ad in particular; I am concerned about hospital advertisements in general. Success rates are statistical information, which is widely and notoriously misunderstood. The overall impression given by an advertisement containing statistical information may vary greatly from its literal content. This is so for two different reasons. First, there is the fallibility of the judgments people make about statistical matters, even when they are being deliberate and reflective.

This problem is well documented; contemporary cognitive psychologists have shown that people typically process statistical information in deeply flawed ways. There is an almost universal tendency to ignore statistically valid base-rate data, even when it is readily available, in the face of atypical, but vivid, anecdotal evidence or powerful visual images. (In the exercise I used, are people misled by the habit of thinking that since 98% is typically an A+, the test must be very good?)

This is a humbling fact about how the human mind works, but a fact nonetheless. If what is deceptive is that which induces, and can be reasonably expected to induce, beliefs that are untrue, then the perils of any essentially statistical advertising may be substantial.*

Second, and perhaps more important, is that advertising is largely a noncognitive interaction between advertiser and consumer. For that reason, it is a mistake to focus too narrowly on the cognitive content of advertising, looking only at the truth of its claims and the validity of its inferences. They may be no more than peripheral to how advertising works. There is a significant cognitive component in much advertising, sometimes conveying valuable information. But the reality of contemporary advertising is

---

* See, for example, *Judgment under Uncertainty: Heuristics and Biases,* ed. Daniel Kahneman, Paul Slovic, and Amos Tversky (Cambridge: Cambridge University Press, 1982), especially "Acts versus Fears: Understanding Perceived Risks," by Paul Slovic, Baruch Fischoff, and Sarah Lichtenstein, pp. 463–89.

that the provision of accurate information to the consumer is often secondary or even absent; paradigmatic of such an information-free ad is one showing an attractive and apparently wholesome person in a beautiful setting smoking a cigarette, with the brand name of the cigarette the only verbal content of the ad.

Many advertisements avoid saying anything false by avoiding the assertion of any propositions whatever. This can be done by limiting the advertisement to visual images; it can also be done, after the fashion of some political speechwriting, by limiting the verbal content to the meaningless. An example of that is an airline advertisement some years ago affirming that "Being first isn't everything, it's the only thing." Or, perhaps it was "Being first isn't the only thing, it's everything." Since neither claim means anything, I can't remember which was the one in the advertisement. (And I certainly can't recall which airline's nonsense it was.) Such claims cannot be false because, lacking cognitive content, they can't be either true or false. But they may play a role in deception, for the routes to deception are not solely cognitive. Our beliefs are determined only in part by rational judgment, just as our decisions are determined only in part by our beliefs.

Should we now regulate health care advertising, beyond the constraints imposed by current barriers to fraud and deception? Any response to this question will presuppose deep commitments about political theory and the proper role of government in relation to the public interest. Government must protect the public interest in various ways through regulation, but the stringency of regulations ought to reflect the degree of risk and the modes of redress that are available, and should not merely reflect the degree to which the behavior in question offends the sensibilities of some people. Not everything deplorable ought to be regulated or prohibited.

Note also the considerable difference between goods and services. Goods are durable in time; even if the complaint is that they have broken or worn out prematurely, what remains can be examined long after the moment of acquisition. Further, manufactured goods admit of sampling techniques that can enhance quality control. Even so, it is often very difficult to obtain redress when one has been victimized by shoddy goods or deceptive advertising in relation to consumer goods. As Lee Weiner said, writing of the Federal Trade Commission's ad substantiation program:

> An individual consumer's injury from deceptive advertising is typically too minor, in economic terms, to justify recourse to the judicial system . . . even when consumers are aware that they have been victimized by fraudulent ad representations, little practical recourse is available.*

Weiner adds that the FTC's effort "to combat deceptive advertisements by eliminating representations that take advantage of the consumer's lack of technical expertise . . . has failed, on almost all counts, to achieve its goals." Yet Weiner was writing of goods, with which substantiation is considerably easier than with professional services.

Who might the victims be of advertising of health care services? We must know that before we can consider what modes of constraint might be appropriate. The most obvious victim is the direct consumer of misrepresented services. Competitors who lose business to the deceptive advertiser also are victimized. But there can be less obvious victims, as well. Identifiable persons depicted in an advertisement can be victims. This could be so, for example, if the facilities of a hospital's psychiatric unit were shown with a recognizable patient inadvertently visible in the background. More commonly, categories of persons exemplified by the individuals in an ad can be victimized; this has surely been the case with many ads depicting women and minority group members in ways that reinforce stereotypical images detrimental to their interests. Women are still the victims of much television advertising that continues to portray them in belittling, demeaning, and humiliating ways. Indeed, children and men are also victimized by such distorted images of women's roles. This victimization is a broadly based social phenomenon, far removed from the level of the direct consumer. In this respect, consider also automobile advertisements which in America have returned to an emphasis on speed, power, and "macho" driving; the results may be—although this would be hard to document—an increased level of carnage on the

---

*"The Ad Substantiation Program: You Can Fool All of the People Some of the Time and Some of the People All of the Time, but Can You Fool the FTC?" *American University Law Review* 30–415 (1981):431.

highways and a corresponding increase in health insurance costs generally. (In Britain, for this reason, automotive advertising is regulated; even in magazine advertisements, the depiction of excessive speed is prohibited.)

A profession, too, may be victimized by the advertising of one of its members, if that ad misrepresents the nature of the profession or causes public opprobrium that is generalized, beyond the individual advertiser, to the image of the profession overall. So doctors and lawyers are properly concerned about advertising that might "give the profession a bad name," and hospitals are rightly concerned about becoming involved in competitive advertising campaigns that can diminish public respect for hospitals as institutions serving the public interest.

But at what level of generality is victimization by advertising the proper object of intervention—that of the direct consumer only, the broader social environment, or something between? This is a question of some complexity; the answer may depend on variable factors such as the level of risk and the available remedies for harms in each kind of circumstance.

To protect against victimizations of all these sorts, diverse constraints, beyond reliance on the good judgment of sponsors, already limit the content of advertising to some extent. A contemplated ad may be rejected because it violates the law, a code or standard of the sponsoring industry or profession, the standards of the advertising agency, or the requirements of the media through which the ad is to be placed. Ads can violate none of these things, however, and still violate standards of taste. Each level of restraint constitutes a protection against violations of certain sorts in behalf of potential victims.

A profession, through its own code of advertising standards, may be centrally concerned with protecting the reputation of that profession, and may forbid advertisements that would be inoffensive to a newspaper. But the newspaper, concerned with the social consequences of the stereotyping reflected in its ads, might reject an advertisement that was not seen as offensive by the professional association.

This is as it should be. The various categories of potential victims of poor advertising constitute interest groups with different, although overlapping, concerns. Those interests are properly protected by different mechanisms, depending on the scope and severity of the harms at issue.

What restraints are needed on the advertising of health care services must be determined piecemeal, along with the development of such advertising, as various types and levels of risk are discerned. Restraint on the part of individual hospitals and their associations should prevent advertisements of the sort I wrote from ever appearing, and individual physicians, possibly restrained by guidelines within their profession, should limit their promotional activity to a forthright and honest presentation of relevant information. But the growing competition for health care dollars may lead to aggressive and unrestrained promotion that will invite new mechanisms of constraint.

An advertisement for a physician in New York inquires, "Psoriasis Sufferers, Why Suffer? 88% cleared!" Reprinted in *Hospital Tribune* (May 16, 1984), it illustrates a point emphasized by the article it accompanies—that medical advertising is on the rise, and will have to be taken into account even by physicians and hospitals hostile to advertising. An adjacent article describes a physician in Milwaukee who budgets $100,000 a year to advertise the services of his four-person clinic, and whose aggressive marketing approach has prompted other physicians to advocate regulation by the profession that would place rigid controls on the content and form of medical advertising. That seems unlikely, in the judgment of an advertising agency professional who specializes in medical accounts, however; he told the newspaper that "The Supreme Court has made it clear that so long as ads are not misleading or fraudulent or do not violate good taste, there is no limit on the content or medium."

Will we see advertisement one day by the Wholesome Hospital? It is too soon to tell. Advertising by the major hospital corporations thus far seems tasteful and restrained. For example, the Hospital Corporation of America took a full page in the October 1984 *Smithsonian* to tell the story of how its newly acquired Navarro Regional Hospital was able to provide care to indigent and uninsured patients because of the innovative establishment of a Health Services Foundation, with funds from the sale of the hospital to HCA, in order to underwrite the costs of care for those not otherwise able to pay their bills. But HCA now controls over 400 hospitals. As it travels around the country—a corporate Pac-man gobbling up little hospitals by the day—in competition with Humana, other for-profit corporations, and the nonprofit sector, will all the competitive gloves stay on? We may yet see advertising that is not demonstrably deceptive by legal standards, yet invites misunderstanding, serving the interests of the competing corporations in a manner that is contrary to the public interest, and increasing the pressure on hospitals like Boston's Beth Israel to participate more assertively in the competition.

This may not occur, but it would be naive to assume that self-restraint, good taste, and dedication to the public good on the part of corporate medicine and individual practitioners will prevent it. It may not be easy to decide how far to go in marketing health care, or what measures, of what degree of severity, will be appropriate to protect the public interest in respect to advertising of hospital services. But considering these matters prospectively may pay dividends later.

At medical grand rounds, the subject is the impact on hospitals of prospective payment plans, which specify revenues in advance. Diagnosis-related groups (DRGs) are one such plan, and they all impose some financial risk on hospitals. The speaker is not an economist, but a physician. The setting is not an administrative meeting, but medical rounds. The subject is medical economics, and the message is sobering.

With fixed rates of reimbursement playing a major role in hospital finances, there is a need to lower the hospital's cost per case. We can reduce the average length of stay, reduce the number of inputs (such as test results) per case, and increase efficiency in other ways. But this can reduce the quality of care and slow the adoption of expensive new treatments, however good they may be. The safeguards of quality are professional norms, careful monitoring, and the spectre of malpractice. But we may need to devise better monitoring systems and measures of patient satisfaction.

There is financial pressure on hospitals to increase their volume, to reduce or eliminate the provision of free care to the indigent, to reduce their unbillable involvement in medical education, and to select those patients whom it is most likely they can treat at low cost in relation to the fixed DRG payments. This suggests avoiding the more seriously ill patients within a particular diagnostic group, and it means avoiding "sinker patients," such as the older patient who recovers more slowly or the patient from lower socioeconomic groups who is likely to have a more complicated recovery.

To increase the occupancy and therefore the efficiency of coronary care units, the speaker notes, a hospital might want to consider advertising on local television.

.9.

LEARNING
MEDICINE
IN THE
"HOUSE OF
GOD"

Medical students, house officers, and attending and staff physicians spend much of their time in hospitals puzzling about what is true. They try to learn what is true about each individual patient, in order to provide suitable treatment. But even knowing what is true of a patient, they can treat competently only if they are also well informed about medicine. So they try to learn what is true in general about diseases and cures.

Medical students are keenly aware of how little knowledge of either kind they have, but they often have yet to understand how fully the battle against ignorance will become a permanent part of their struggles. As medical students, they perhaps think that learning medicine is what they must do to become doctors. As doctors, they will realize that learning medicine is something they must continue unendingly to do in order to be doctors.

There are three main reasons why physicians at all levels of experience know less than they wish they knew. First, too much is unknown about health and illness generally. Second, too much is known about health and illness generally. Third, some of what is crucial to know is unknowable.

What is understood about the origins and processes of illness has increased immensely in our lifetime. The successes of modern medicine are largely based on that understanding. But most of what we would like to know about health and illness remains to be discovered. We can transplant kidneys to keep patients alive on dialysis, but we do not know how to prevent kidneys from failing. We can alleviate pain in most cases, but we do not know how to reverse or halt painful degenerative processes. We can often save the lives of seriously damaged newborns, but we cannot prevent congenital illness. And so on.

We have conquered several diseases, and in that medical science can take great pride. But many more remain as unmet challenges, and the list of such challenges, as AIDS has taught us so well, can grow as well as shrink. Despite our astonishing progress in medical understanding, what we do not know far exceeds what we have learned about the complex vulnerabilities of the human organism. This first source of ignorance limits every doctor's ability to treat patients. It fuels medical research, and makes it necessary for doctors to remain students of medicine throughout their professional lives as new information flows daily from that research.

At the same time, what is already known about diseases and how they can be treated is far more than any single human mind can master. Every physician is therefore partially ignorant not merely in not knowing what is as yet undiscovered, but also in not knowing some large portion of what has already been learned by medical science.

Consider the use of prescription drugs as an illustration of this second source of ignorance. The *Physicians' Desk Reference*—the PDR, as it is known—is an annually revised compendium of information about drugs currently available for therapeutic use in the United States. (Although intended for health care providers, it is properly a part of any home reference library, since it supplies much more information about the risks, benefits, and uses of each drug than patients are typically given by their doctors.) The 1988 edition, weighing nearly six pounds, comprises 2354 large-format (8½" x 11") pages. The index of prescription drugs by brand and generic names goes on for seventeen four-column pages, filled with tiny print! Spring and Fall supplements are published each year to bring the volume up to date between its annual revisions—another 143 pages for 1988. How could anyone reasonably be expected to master even that large portion of such a mass of information that is directly relevant to a particular medical specialty? How can any physician help but be uncertain about the proper use of at least some of the available drugs?

Recognizing the impossibility of such mastery, health care providers increasingly look to computers to reduce the uncertainty caused by the volume and complexity of medical information. One good example is a project at Stanford some years ago. Physicians were free to prescribe drugs as they saw fit for their hospitalized patients. A computerized record system in the hospital pharmacy, updated with current information about the effects and interactions of all the drugs in use, then checked each prescription against the patient's record to detect any possible adverse reactions or contraindications in light of that patient's individual history of allergies, other physiological characteristics, and other medications. Most of the prescriptions written each day—well over 95%—were approved by the computer without question. Even among those flagged as raising questions, most—but not quite all—were appropriate, all things considered, as the best available option despite the apparent risk. Still, with 900 prescriptions a day written on average during one year of the project, even that very small error rate yielded several instances a day of prescriptions that were revised because the computer check led to the judgment that they were not in the patients' best interest.

Such effective computer systems are very expensive; this limits the extent to which they can reduce the uncertainty that besets physicians. Also, as new drugs and new understandings of old drugs are an on-going part of medical progress, it takes constant effort to supply such systems with the latest information. In principle, a national drug data bank could be created, providing all hospitals with an electronic enhancement of the PDR, helping the hospital evaluate its use of drugs with information that is current and complete.

If that were done, the volume of medical information of other kinds relevant to any patient's case would still challenge the mind of even the most brilliant physician. In any event, it takes no account of the vast range of uncertainty about what has or has not been established by pharmacological research, as reflected in continuing debates in the medical literature about the adequacy of drug studies and the various interpretations to which they are open.

The third source of ignorance is even harder to defeat. As Alasdair MacIntyre and I have written elsewhere, there is an essential fallibility in medical judgment because medicine is a practical discipline aimed at doing good for specific individuals, no two completely alike. Much of what a doctor needs to know in treating a particular patient is not general medical or physiological information, but is specific to that patient—which is why the medical history is so important to clinical examination.

Some of the necessary information is available via that medical history, but in most cases additional evidence about the patient is needed. Much of that additional information is now gained from tests, such as blood tests or EKGs, and from imaging procedures, such as magnetic resonance imaging or X rays. These tests are a kind of research—research about what is true of the specific patient. But the fragility of the human subject limits the extent to which that research can yield answers. The pursuit of knowledge about the patient can be dangerously invasive, so physicians must sometimes proceed to treatment without having as much detailed information as they would prefer. After all, if the tests and examinations kill the patient, even the most exquisite knowledge of what was wrong is little comfort.

Each treatment is the treatment of a specific individual about whom there is always partial uncertainty. Each therapeutic intervention is, for that reason, also a kind of research. It is not research aimed primarily at a better general understanding of medical knowledge (although it can contribute to that understanding.) It is an experiment to see if *this* treatment will help *this* patient *this* time. So much is unknown about any particular patient that trial and error is necessarily a part of even the best medical care most of the time. If this essential uncertainty in the art of medicine were more broadly understood (and publicly acknowledged by physicians), there might be less litigation over disappointing outcomes—to the greater benefit of us all.

As a New York State Department of Health study (*Monitoring Health Care Quality*) reported in 1988, four-fifths of adverse medical outcomes are due to factors other than medical negligence. This is reflected in the outcomes of malpractice claims, most of which are closed without payment to the plaintiff. Yet even a successful defense is very costly in legal fees, time, and distraction. These costs, added to the judgments in successful litigations (over $122 million in New York State in 1983, the most recent year of the study), are reflected in the very high price of malpractice insurance and, in turn, in the costs of medical care—which might be considerably lower given greater public understanding of the inherent limitations of medical understanding.

This third source of ignorance is also a barrier to developing computerized diagnostic protocols. A computer program can only use the information that is available; what is unknown and unknowable about a patient will remain unknown even if a sophisticated diagnostic protocol exists. Some physicians nonetheless look to computers, and especially to "expert systems" computers, to integrate what is known more fully than humans can on their own, and to provide diagnostic and therapeutic guidance, thereby reducing the effects of the uncertainty that pervades medicine. Others are less sanguine, arguing that experienced clinical judgment will remain the central ingredient in good medical care and that programmed protocols not only won't help, but will constrain the beneficial exercise of such judgment.

All these sources of uncertainty are part of the reality of medicine and would exist no matter what the structure of medicine as a social institution and no matter what the competence and dedication of physicians. In addition, physicians are beset by the full variety of human frailties, and medicine is a social institution limited by cultural realities. Fatigue and anxiety, frustration and anger, bias and distraction can also be a part of the reality of medical practice.

See, for instance, such stories as "The Use of Force" and "Old Doc Rivers" by William Carlos Williams, the physician-author whose compelling portrayals of doctors reveal complex blends of competence and crudeness, compassion and arrogance, anger toward patients and commitment to their interests. Economic and social conditions can also limit the possibilities of care. Yet, amidst all this uncertainty and constraint, medical students and physicians must learn how to function as doctors and how to treat specific patients, one by one. How, I wondered, do they do it?

It is late May, the first weekend following my arrival at the hospital. Settled in at my studio apartment on Commonwealth Avenue, I welcome a bit of time that is less intensely scheduled than during the week. I turn to a novel I have been carrying around for weeks, but haven't begun. At least a dozen people have told me to read it, especially since I am going to be in residence at Beth Israel Hospital. All I know is that it is about an intern.

The paperback copy of The House of God *has been around the house for a couple of years, since someone gave it, already dog-eared, to one of my children. It has obviously been read by quite a few before me. The author is Samuel Shem, M.D.; the book is ostensibly about contemporary hospital care.*

Published in 1978, the story is set in an urban, Jewish hospital affiliated with a highly prestigious medical school. The narrator, Roy Basch, tells of his year as an intern in the House of God—a year of deprivation, degradation, pain, bumbling, acting-out with immense immaturity, deteriorating interpersonal relationships, and increasing cynicism. As I read, I see that it is an unrestrainedly self-indulgent book, full of rage, exaggerated stereotypes, and savage satire too crudely written and leniently edited to do much damage, yet with a macabre humor that, in places, is undeniably funny. Its portrayal of the almost uninterrupted sexual adventures of the house officers and nurses is utterly vulgar and devoid of the subtlety that might make for erotic appeal. It paints a picture of a hospital run jointly by Kafka, the Marquis de Sade, and the Marx Brothers. And yet, I read on. The House of God, it quickly becomes apparent, is (as a reviewer in the Medical Tribune *had put it in 1978) "the scarcely veiled prestigious Boston Beth Israel Hospital," where the pseudonymous Shem, now practicing psychiatry, had been an intern.*

It is early in July. As I enter the cafeteria at lunchtime, the chief of one of the medical departments draws me into a private room at the back of the main dining area. There, over lunch, he greets the new crop of residents. He emphasizes that the challenge of the future is in their hands, and that they are a superbly qualified group, having been chosen in a highly selective process. He acknowledges that the program they have entered is very demanding both physically and emotionally. There are less demanding programs, he concedes, but reminds them that they have chosen to come to this one. They can expect to suffer from nervousness, Autumn depression, and sleep disorders, he warns.

I am paying close attention. Yet, in the back of my mind I hear the voice of Mabel, Major-General Stanley's daughter, as she sings a song of encouragement to the assembled police in Gilbert and Sullivan's The Pirates of Penzance, *urging them on into battle against the dreaded pirates:*

> *Go ye heros, go to glory,*
> *Though you die in combat gory,*
> *Ye shall live in song and story.*
> *Go to immortality!*
> *Go to death and go to slaughter;*
> *Die, and every Cornish daughter*
> *With her tears your grave shall water.*
> *Go, ye heroes, go and die!*

These new doctors are in for plenty of gore, death, and what will surely seem like combat. The glory, such as it is, comes later. I hope they all survive.

Now the remarks turn to the constant challenges the residents will face, and they are especially admonished to be vigorous in pursuit of permissions to conduct autopsies. "There are many surprises at autopsy," they are told. "It's the best way to find the sources of major errors." A bit late, I think, from some points of view, but probably essential all the same.

Later, I meet very briefly with these newcomers. I ask how many of them have read a book called The House of God. *Nearly all their hands shoot up.*

The reviewer in the *Medical Tribune* had also said that "Everyone who has been a house officer, recently or in the receding past, will identify with the novel." And *Publishers Weekly*, describing the book as a "mordantly funny, brilliantly ironic and iconoclastic," account of an intern "trying to survive the incredible tensions,

fear and crippling fatigue of the first year of medical practice,"
claimed that "The picture Shem gives us of hospital policies and
politics will shock most readers, but those in the medical profession will recognize the scenes as starkly truthful."

I had wondered about how medicine is learned and taught in
Boston's Beth Israel. Shem's book offered one answer in some
detail. Implausible though it seemed to me, it had obviously
captured the attention of a large public. Something about it
seemed credible to the point that a reviewer could use a phrase like
"starkly truthful." If Shem did not portray a reality, at least he had
portrayed a perceived reality.

He had also, I suspected, captured an important source of anxiety in the house officers. Having finished medical school, they
were now doctors. But the context of uncertainty around them
revealed that doctors though they may be, they would always
remain students of medicine. Trained for years, as premedical and
medical students, in learning large amounts of factual information, they were now embarked on a career in which many of the
facts they most wanted were elusive, and the ones they had were
inadequate. After a decade of being rewarded for memorizing
facts, they had left certainty behind; the world of judgment and
probability was now the world they inhabited, and lives were at
stake. Perhaps they could not help seeing that world as somewhat
mad; perhaps that is part of why Shem's book became a basic text
for so many of them. I had finished the book, laughing robustly
here, wincing there, and mainly just slogging on toward the end,
with increasing interest in comparing the real Beth Israel with
Shem's "House of God."

Some of what I subsequently saw made me more sympathetic in
retrospect to Shem's sense of the bizarre. The late-night resuscitation of the dying woman was a scene that could easily have come
from the book. Poor old Sophie, who just screamed and screamed
in the dialysis unit, and the old man who chanted "Doctor Doctor
Doctor Doctor," could well have been among Shem's characters.
And surely I saw grinding fatigue among the young doctors, even
as I experienced it when I briefly shared their on-call schedule. So
several of the ingredients of Shem's portrayal have some basis in
fact. The most striking difference, however, is that in *The House of
God* the prevailing climate is one of competition, cynicism, and ill

will, whereas in the real world, despite its imperfections, the prevailing climate is one of cooperation, dedication, and good will.

That is not to say that house officer training isn't a miserable ordeal. Those I spoke to, without exception, believed that the rigors of their servitude were more nearly the product of tradition and economics than any pedagogical justification. The senior physicians were more divided; one, a gentle, supportive internist who was very conscientious in the mentoring of his apprentices, said, "It teaches them to put patient care interests first, no matter how one feels. That's a crucial lesson one never forgets." But the credibility of that view remains a matter of debate.

In 1981, Norman Cousins engendered substantial controversy with "Internship: Preparation or Hazing?," an opinion piece in the *Journal of the American Medical Association* in which he concluded that "the custom of overworking interns . . . is inconsistent with the public interest" and is not "worthy of the tradition of medicine." The journal received "an avalanche of thoughtful commentary" in reply, with the defenders of the traditional internship slightly outnumbering Cousin's supporters.

If the matter divides the medical profession, however, with those who have been through that *rite d'passage* slightly favoring its retention, the issue has engaged the attention of many outside the halls of medical training who are not so sympathetic to it. In New York State, for example, new legislation restricts the extent to which hospitals can require house officers to serve without sleep, and imposes minimum weekly periods of time off. Since July 1989, house officers have been limited (except in very small hospitals) to no more than twelve consecutive hours of duty in emergency settings, may not be scheduled for more than twenty-four consecutive hours of work, and must not work more than an average of eighty hours a week over any four-week period. That may seem like scant solace to residents, but it does represent a substantial improvement in their working conditions, especially as the law also requires that they be granted at least eight hours off between assignments and at least one twenty-four hour period off each week (the statute is 10NYCRR405.4(b)(6)). Implementing these reforms may well protect the public interest by reducing errors of judgment or performance due to fatigue, but it also reduces the low cost medical labor force in teaching hospitals, and therefore is another upward pressure on the costs of medical care.

Returning to my office, I find a draft manuscript by Robert Levin, a psychiatrist in the hospital. He has noted on it, "I'd appreciate your thoughts when you have an opportunity to read this." The title is "Housestaff Training Stress." I read it eagerly, and schedule a conversation with Dr. Levin. The essay discusses the nature, origins, and effects of stress in house officers; some of the behavior described in the draft sounds very like that of the interns in Shem's novel. We discuss the draft and the issues it raises, especially the impact on young doctors of the transition from medical student to house officer, which requires their coming to see more clearly the negatives of the profession as they confront the need to deal from positions of responsibility with the distasteful and the tragic.

Dr. Levin's article appeared in *General Hospital Psychiatry* (10, 114–121, 1988) under the title "Beyond 'The Men of Steel': The Origins and Significance of House Staff Training Stress." Citing public concern about the effects of staff stress on the quality of patient care, Levin notes with favor the new regulations in New York State before concluding:

> Senior physicians need to change their values and role responsibilities in order to acknowledge the significance of training stress. . . . It should be the professional and personal obligation of physician educators to recognize and address training stress openly. . . . Medical educators have responsibilities toward their house officers who are also their students and colleagues. . . . We should promote good training and the appropriate growth of trainees as physicians and as individuals. The teaching of good doctoring—of patients, of colleagues, of oneself—should begin in the house staff years.

Whether or not the structure and conditions of work for house officers evolves into something different, more healthful, and more humane, one feature of their experience is sure to remain constant. Medical work in a hospital is intensely interactive. Doctors spend much of their time talking—to nurses, patients, and one another. There is little time, place, or occasion for quiet reflection. The talk is sometimes general, and often about a particular case, with participants from various specialties. Sometimes it is in a structured setting such as grand rounds or a particular specialty's case conferences. Sometimes it is in the halls or stairway—especially during the frequent, extremely long waits for elevators. (These are excellent environments for eavesdropping, which provides a rich sense of fabric of life in an institution.) Typically, wherever it occurs, there is a mix of participants and listeners including medical students, house officers, and senior physicians. It is in the midst of this immersion in talk, of the give and take of constant questioning, probing, conjecturing, that the learning of medicine goes on.

I arrive a few minutes early for the daily case conference on the unit. A medical student is there, too, and we begin to chat about his program and his ambitions. The medical students' dormitory is simply dreadful, he reports. "Why live there?," I ask.

"It's an awful, narrow, intense atmosphere. Everybody has the same stresses and the same problems; it's a really artificial world. But I suppose it is useful to have a lot of people around who are studying the same things. And expensive as it is at $300 a month, it's a lot cheaper than anything else around here. I will have $60,000 in debts when I graduate as it is."

We talk a bit more, about his college days and his ambitions. "I suppose I'd like to go into medical research. But it's out of the question. I can't even consider it. With the debts I have for my education, I have to start earning some real money as soon as I can. It wasn't easy for my parents when I was in college. They don't have much, but they helped me a lot. I can't ask them to help me now, but I'm mortgaging my future by being here."

A visiting medical student from Europe says that he, too, is interested in medical research. But for him, there is no financial barrier. Medical education in his country is publicly supported, so he will not carry a great burden of debt when he finishes his training. He will be able to afford not to let his choices be dominated by financial considerations.

At one time, learning medicine was a highly prestigious goal, eagerly sought by a large proportion of the nation's brightest students. They were admired and envied if they gained access to medical school, thereby embarking on the path to an honored, well-rewarded, and gratifying career. Like teaching, nursing, or social work, it offered the great satisfactions of service to others. Unlike them, however, it also offered the affluence of a successful career in business. No wonder it was so eagerly sought.

Now, fewer good students are attracted to that path. The high cost of medical education in the United States has been cited as one of the major factors accounting for the sharp decline in applications to medical school, which dropped by 31% from 1977 to 1987 (from over 40,000 to just over 28,000). Medical school admissions officers express concern that applicants may soon be accepted who would have been judged unqualified a decade ago, and that a shortage of physicians may ensue. There are other factors, as well; the *Chronicle of Higher Education* (June 15, 1988) cites the increasing desire of young people to earn money quickly; the widespread, but controversial, perception that an overabundance of doctors will limit professional opportunity; and growing awareness of "the negative aspects of medicine, including the high cost of malpractice insurance and the increasingly bureaucratic nature of the medical profession." And it doesn't help that medical education is perceived as intellectually sterile and medical training as inhumane.

Despite these problems, many bright students still enter medicine, and those who go to Boston's Beth Israel as house officers have been among the most successful in medical school. They learn medicine, along with their mentors and the Harvard medical students on clinical rotations, through observation, guided participation in diagnostic and treatment procedures, and constant conversation about many aspects of medical care.

At the surgical chief's rounds, the topic is surgical treatment of pancreatitis. I learn that in Trinidad, scorpion stings are the most common cause of pancreatitis. I never did much like the look of scorpions; I'm happy to have a better reason than aesthetic prejudice for continuing to avoid them.

The surgeons discuss some data that suggest success at relieving the pain of pancreatitis by surgical means. But, one of them points out, if the pain of pancreatitis is self-limiting, the data showing relief of pain are not significant and the surgical pro-

cedure is not important. The surgeon cautions that the operation is perhaps done "to get there before the pain goes away on its own." But the evidence is inconclusive about whether the pain is self-limiting.

What if I run into a scorpion all the same, and end up with pancreatitis, or get it some other way? Would I now be best advised to rule surgery out as being of unconfirmed benefit? What questions would I ask a consulting surgeon, now that I have seen their own uncertainty? What would I be able to make of their answers? Am I better off for knowing about their skepticism?

At the weekly medical management conference, the chief resident presents a case for the consideration of the audience—primarily house officers, medical students, staff, and attending physicians in internal medicine. The patient is a 29-year-old woman with obesity and exertional fatigue; she was admitted through the emergency room because of dyspnea (substantial distress in breathing) and loss of consciousness. She was on no medication and there is no family history of cardiac or pulmonary disease. "Dyspnea and fatigue. What are the first things you think about?" asks the chief resident.

"Heart and lungs," replies an intern. The chronic buzz of low-level conversation in the room increases, as the discussion turns to the variety of ailments that could account for the presenting problem. The open door to the rear is in constant use, as doctors come late, leave early, or answer pages.

"How would you begin the workup?" asks the chief. The air is thick with the names of medical tests—X rays, blood gas analysis, echo-cardiography, and more. Now, the results of some of the woman's tests are revealed. There is right ventricular enlargement; there is pulmonary hypertension. "What can account for pulmonary hypertension?" There are at least a hundred possibilities. I hear mention of several as "consistent with the findings." No one speaks in terms of the cause; no one even says "probably."

The chest X ray, another clue, is revealed. "Scleroderma?" ventures one contestant; "atrial septal defect?" offers another. I find myself thinking of a television game show until the grim truth dispels that image; the woman's heart is damaged beyond repair and is worsening rapidly. "This disease does not present itself clinically until the end stage," the chief resident explains, "and it is very hard to pick up early." A senior physician is speaking now: "We must deal with the reality that this is a very serious disease with a poor prognosis. She must be advised to get her affairs in order."

"What about a transplant?" asks another doctor. She would need a heart-lung transplant, the senior physician explains. It is a desperate option, and the odds are long against her being selected. Her packet will go to three transplant centers, but with little chance of success. A young doctor asks about an additional study that might be done; the senior physician replies: "Time is so precious for such a patient, I am reluctant to bring her back for another invasive study. She's 30 years old. That's why nobody lets them die, because they're 30 years old. They get flogged half the time."

The uncertainty that is so common in medical diagnosis and treatment has led some to the hope that computer-based information systems can reduce the variability of practice and its reliance on intuitive and fallible clinical judgment, by compensating for the natural limitations of human memory and powers of analysis. Computers already play a role, at least on a pilot basis, in taking a thorough medical history, determining the most probable diagnosis, selecting the optimal drugs, and deciding on the most appropriate treatment. But it is dangerous to expect computers to remedy all the deficiencies of medical judgment. Recall the story of Mr. S, who sought to have his ankle examined, and, as a "major donor," was asked on admission about the donation of his organs. Despite its humor, the story highlights a growing concern in hospitals—which is why it was taken seriously by the hospital administrators.

In many fields, such as the development of weapon systems, costs are notoriously underestimated, while performance chronically lags far behind even the most solemn promises. Computer technology, however, has outstripped all but the most wildly optimistic expectations. The contrast is so striking that we can easily be misled into overestimating its capacity to eliminate the need for human judgment and thereby to eliminate errors due to uncertainty and the fallibility of that judgment. But computers and the software systems that animate them are human artifacts. As health care becomes increasingly dependent on computers, used not just to store and transmit information, but to analyze and interpret it and to generate recommendations about what should be done, the inherent limitations of software design provide new sources of uncertainty and surprise. Although computers can greatly assist our efforts to improve the quality of health care, they can not eliminate uncertainty, error, or the need for judgment.

Learning to improve the quality of care is not just a challenge for physicians, of course, but for all who deal with patients. The nursing staff is particularly sensitive to the importance of their impact on the patients; their relationship to patients is more intimate and continuous than that of doctors, and the scope of their concerns is in some ways more broad.

Beth Israel's nursing staff is renowned nationally for an extraordinarily high quality of patient care, based on the concept of Primary Nursing—which makes each admitted patient the responsibility of a particular nurse throughout the patient's hospitalization. Other nurses will be involved as the shifts change, but the planning and oversight of the patient's care remains the responsibility of the primary nurse. At Boston's Beth Israel, nurses typically enjoy the respect and cooperation of the attending physicians, and function with a higher degree of autonomy and responsibility than nurses in most other settings. And they, too, have grand rounds.

A panel of nurses has been discussing the effect of DRGs on the nurses' relationship with patients, pointing out that care has been moved to "fast-forward." Then the primary presenter turns to the main topic of the day, the impact on nursing of high technology in the cardiac care unit.

"We are dealing with more technology and sicker patients," she points out. Nurses are increasingly involved in invasive procedures at the bedside, such as Swan-Ganz lines and angioplasty. She speaks of the "sense of invested self" that the nurses have in regard to their patients, noting that with the pressure to move patients through more quickly, nurses sometimes have battles to

fight in the patients' behalf, and, in the fast pace that results, "You sometimes need to call in the head nurse or others to help fight your battles."

The role that nurses now play can be frightening; it can take a special effort to overcome one's own anxiety to provide the comfort that a patient needs in a critical situation. But there is frustration involved in working with those doctors who impede the nurses' close relationship with the patients, treating the nurses as "PPOs—professional package openers."

In the Emergency Room, patients are seen briefly. But the primary nursing approach applies there as well, the speaker explains, and the key issue is accountability. Even in the ER, one nurse is accountable for one patient regardless of duration, and that accountability includes "assessing nursing care needs, referrals to home care, arranging for visiting nurses as necessary, and providing continuity for repeaters. There must be a coordinated care plan similar to those that are written on the floors."

I hadn't thought about repeaters being a problem; emergency rooms are where one goes in an emergency, which by their very nature are rare, I thought. But I listen and learn, as the speaker describes a patient who "came in just about every other day for four years. He became a real management problem. But a group discussion led to a coordinated care plan which he accepted. He's around just as much, but he isn't a management problem now."

After some discussion of the need for follow-up of emergency room patients, she concludes on a cautionary note: "There's a constant testing of limits with a lot of the interns and a few other doctors. One of them actually said to me, 'There are two domains, the doctor's and the nurse's. You stay there and there will be no problem.' But I told him, 'No, there's all this area in between.'"

If that intern listened and understood, he learned two important points about the art of medicine. One is that grey areas abound, and the rigid sort of categorical thinking he displayed, which is common among medical students, can be an impediment to good care. He might also have realized that young doctors stand to learn much about medical care from the nurses who play such an important role in providing and monitoring it. The house officer who, albeit brilliant, arrogantly sees the nurse as an instrument for the implementation of his decisions is not an unknown type even at Boston's Beth Israel. But those who seek to become the best clinicians they can be will welcome wisdom where they find it, and the nurses have a lot of it to offer. And they seek to deepen that wisdom as they can.

In the orthopedic unit, the nurses gather for a meeting with the hospital chaplain. He has come at their request to discuss an issue that puzzles them; they want to know more about the dietary laws that govern the choices made by their orthodox Jewish patients. As I meet these nurses, I realize that in this Jewish hospital, I have not yet met a Jewish nurse. Although there are a few in the profession, nursing is like banking or aviation in being an over- whelmingly Christian profession, and in that respect is unlike medicine, social work, or teaching, in which there are large Jewish representations.

The Rabbi discusses the significance of ethnic differences and practices to the various kinds of patients in the hospital, explain- ing that autonomy with respect to diet is of particular importance as an aspect of life over which the patient can retain some valuable control. Errors in the provision of food emphasize their loss of control as patients, which is why such errors can be so upsetting. Since orthodox Jewish food laws are similar to those of the Jehovah's Witnesses, he continues, Witnesses often order kosher food in the hospital. But it is bad for people with hypertension; the salt used in koshering meat to draw out the blood is bad for those with a low-sodium diet, so their meat must be soaked in water to reduce the salt content. And all dietary laws are suspended for Jewish patients if necessary in the interest of saving life.

The nurses are puzzled by a particular case. Mrs. G, 88, has ordered kosher brisket of beef for dinner, but has also asked for ice cream. She seems a little confused, and the nurses know that the orthodox will not have both meat and milk at the same meal. If she is orthodox, her order may be an accident, but the nurses do not want to seem to criticize her by asking about it. Neither do they want her to be upset when the meal arrives. The Rabbi explains that people sometimes interpret dietary laws in very idiosyn- cratic ways. Perhaps she is not strictly kosher, but just prefers kosher meat. Her order might have been entirely intentional. But it could be a confusion, so it is worth going over it with her, just to confirm that it is what she intended.

He goes on to describe the cultural differences he has perceived in the hospital. Jewish patients and their families are generally more demanding and assertive, wanting to take an active part in the management of their cases. Italians, largely Catholic, are expressive, but more passively accept what occurs. Other cultures, especially some Protestants, fight against being expressive, and may be terrified or upset without being able to reveal it. Oriental families often have such a strong desire to take care of their own that even the fact of hospitalization can be felt as symbolizing a failure of the family. Occasionally, a family's overreaction can even make it hard to reintegrate the patient into the family following the hospitalization. To provide the best care, the nurses must discover the needs of each patient; it may help to be alert to these cultural differences, which can mask a patient's real concerns.

Although there is a critical shortage of nurses nationally, Boston's Beth Israel remains a desirable and well-supported environment for nursing in which positions are eagerly sought. The nursing program, widely admired and constantly visited by delegations from other hospitals, is unique despite many efforts to replicate it elsewhere. The reason doubtless lies not in the formal structure and policies that define that program and which could easily be replicated, but in the institutional culture that sustains it. Perhaps that culture has its roots in the core values and original mission of the Mount Sinai Hospital Association in 1901, or in the particular ethos of Jewish traditions of respect and caring as they are manifested in this environment. In any event, the hospital enjoys a reputation as a desirable context of care, in which the three constituencies of nurses, doctors, and patients interact with an unusual degree of regard for mutual concerns.

Its reputation for sensitivity to patients is reflected in a classic story, told to me by Stanley Taub.

An elderly woman, becoming ill while her son was away from Boston, was taken to another Harvard teaching hospital—one with a superb reputation for important research and excellent care. The next day he rushed to her side, and she demanded immediate transfer to the Beth Israel Hospital. "Why?" asked the son. "Is there a problem with your doctor?

"I can't complain," she replied.

"Is there a problem with the room? The room looks all right to me," he continued.

"I can't complain," she answered.

"Is it the food? Is the food bad?"

"I can't complain," she said once again.

"Then why do you want to go to the Beth Israel?" he asked in frustration.

"There," she explained, "I can complain."

It is not only patients, however, who can complain. So can the doctors.

I accompany a surgeon looking in on several of his post-operative patients late in the day. They are all doing well, and there are no complications. We finish the rounds and head down to pathology. On the way, he tells me that he goes to examine the tissues from every one of his surgical patients, without exception. It is so important, he explains, because the findings are so often different from what was predicted. But, he complains, the younger surgeons these days just won't do it.

Today, he is concerned about a patient who had a region of her stomach with no motility. "It just wouldn't empty," he explains. That section of the stomach has been surgically removed now, and there should be no further problem. "But why was there a problem in the first place? Was it some sort of auto-immune phenomenon?" Not knowing, he is frustrated and discontent.

The pathology laboratory is bright and spotlessly clean. We examine a slide of tissue, less than twelve microns thick, through a microscope that accommodates several viewers. The stained slide looks to me like an image in a kaleidoscope, but it has significance to the surgeon and the pathologist. They discuss what they see for a few minutes, and we head back toward the door.

On the way, I ask the pathologist a question. "How often do the results in pathology show that some aspect of a case was misun-

derstood or misdiagnosed beforehand? Is that a common situation?"

"Every day," he replies, "every single day."

The passion of this surgeon for complete understanding is unusual and exemplary, and his critical remarks about other surgeons reflect the fact that he holds them to the highest possible standard of performance. That surgeons are a breed apart is a common view, even among surgeons, although they do not readily accept the notorious stereotype. The traditional view holds that surgeons are tough, precise, and cold—possessed, like astronauts with the right stuff, of a macho swagger, an air of superiority, and contempt for the "soft" specialties—which is to say, all the others. That image is not at all fair, but it is not all fantasy, either.

Saturday at 8 A.M. the surgeons gather to discuss the week's "complications." Since it is the weekend, the day's work starts later than usual; during the week they have been at the hospital for hours by 8:00 o'clock. This week, there are twenty-one cases on the agenda of the "Mortality and Morbidity Conference." Each case is listed on the agenda along with the name of the surgeon who handled it. There's no hint here of the delicacy that leads to presenting cases anonymously in the OBGYN rounds. Among themselves, the surgeons are as blunt as their scalpels are sharp.

The discussion of the first case is reasonably orderly, despite the disruption of late arrivals, the distraction of construction noise from outside the room, and the buzz of conversation about the case even while it is being presented. By the second case, the order diminishes, as afterthoughts about the first case are unhesitatingly expressed as if the second case had not been presented. One surgeon seems to have been thinking so hard about the first case that he has not noticed the introduction of the second; suddenly he has an insight, and blurts it out from his seat in the audience. Someone responds, and the discussion then glides back to the second case. But I see this only in retrospect; the pace is fast and the vocabulary strange to me, and there is a high level of interruption and of incomplete sentences, so it is hard to tell which case any given remark is about.

Among the first eight cases of complications, two are attributed to errors in diagnosis—one in four. Discussion of the ninth case focuses on an X ray. "We can't distinguish between diverticulitis and a cancer," one of the surgeons explains. There is general agreement about the ambiguity of the images on the screen before us. The surgeon responsible for the case describes what he did "in the end," to which another snaps "which is what you should have done in the first place."

"He's doing well now," responds the first surgeon, and a third asserts, "You were lucky." So, I presume, is the patient, who has now survived not just illness, but ambiguity, uncertainty, mis-diagnosis, treatment, and complications.

The surgeons press on in their quest for a better understanding of their art, and they press one another hard. One makes a statement about the duration of post-operative anticoagulants; another challenges, "You made that statement, but do you have solid evidence for that?" A new X ray is on the screen now, and the discussion turns to the difficulty of distinguishing gas in the venous system from gas in the biliary system. Half an hour here is enough to dispel any thought that diagnosis is a science or that the latest imaging and testing techniques eliminate the need for interpretation, judgment, and even educated guesses about what is going on with a patient.

Halfway through the list of cases, a surgeon acknowledges that he could have figured out a puzzling case sooner: "The thing that should have tipped me off is that she was more comfortable sitting up." That's the sort of thing a surgeon has to know, no matter how well he or she can read the tests and pictures, and this surgeon is taking some heat now for overlooking it.

Much of the discussion centers on post-operative care, and the surgeons make no secret of the fact that they see it as often perilous to turn a patient over to a nonsurgeon. "When you talk about chest tubes in a medical service, it's impending disaster," one complains. "To follow the patient, you have to check the tubes twice a day to verify that they are working, and the doctors on medicine just won't do it." The theme of surgical superiority is woven into the discussion; I have already heard complaints about two other specialties—of one that "They always want to stick the joints," and of another that "They needle-biopsy everything in sight. They have a new toy, and they're using it on everything in sight."

But the complaining is clearly not an advocacy of more surgery. In fact, the complaint is often that unnecessary surgery results from inferior diagnostic judgment, or that the benefit of surgery is undermined by inferior post-operative care. These surgeons are hard on others, but they are hardest on themselves, and they take pride in the fact, as they see it, that they are much harder on themselves than the other specialties are.

It is clear that the techniques of surgery are not completely well-defined, despite the public image of "surgical precision." Discussing incisional hernias, a surgeon says "If somebody can figure out a better way to fix these things, we'd like to hear about it." Discussing a different case, a surgeon describes an innovative procedure he used on a case that presented troublesome surprises in the operating room; an astonished colleague comments, "You did that on a human?"

We near the end of the agenda. A patient has had an "angry" wound infection following surgery. But there was no fever, explains the surgeon, so the infection was not detected quickly. That is a very unusual situation, he suggests.

His colleagues react with incredulity: "That may be covering some tracks."

"It could easily have been detected earlier if it had been looked at."

"Your retrospectoscope is terrific!"

At 9:30, we reach the end of the time and the agenda. In ninety minutes, we have covered twenty-one cases, of which six have involved some sort of misdiagnosis.

These sessions, occurring in every specialty and involving staff at every level of experience, are a regular part of life in the hospital. Of course, there are differences in style and approach among the various specialties. For example, the surgeons take pride in the fact that they discuss every case in which something has gone awry, and they sometimes tend to see the internists, who discuss only a case or two in a comparable session, as superficial in comparison. Yet the surgeons, setting a brisk pace, spent on average just four and a half minutes on each case they discussed on the day I joined them. The internists, on the other hand, take pride in the fact that they discuss their selected cases in depth, spending as much as an hour on a single case, exploring its ramifications thoroughly. So they sometimes tend to see the surgeons as superficial in comparison.

Physicians do take pride in their own specialties, and function within specialty-specific subcultures that color their perceptions of and attitudes toward the others around them. But the kind and extent of mutual hostility Shem portrays is a fantasy. Of course there are fatigue, frustration, shortness of temper, errors in judgment, and stubbornness from time to time. But the essential spirit of the culture, which is what Shem thoroughly misses, is one of striving to perform at a higher level of quality in the provision of medical care, working with one another cooperatively to teach and learn on a daily basis. Still, there is plenty of room for improvement.

Jay Katz, in his important book *The Silent World of Doctor and Patient* (1984), properly laments the lack of adequate conversation between physicians and patients. A major cause of that inadequacy, he explains, is the physician's discomfort with the various dimensions of uncertainty that pervade medicine. Perhaps that same discomfort also partly explains the gaps in the kinds of conversation that go on within medicine. Were it left to me to set the conversational agenda in the hospital, there would be much more discussion between senior doctors and their junior colleagues, about their frustrations, fears, uncertainties, and the stress that results; among the various medical subcultures, about their differences and their commonalities; and even among individual physicians who too often live in the silent world of the doctor, because of a lack of time and of encouragement to be reflective and open about their deepest uncertainties and anxieties. The unending challenge of learning medicine should include a place for unending learning about oneself, but doctors are often too immersed in their own professional lives to reflect on them. Highlighting and legitimizing that agenda could enrich the learning of medicine at every level.

It is a weekend evening at the home of one of the staff physicians. As the guests gather for dinner, I meet another physician who reports on a conversation he has recently heard between two other staff doctors.

"Did you see that that ethics guy has arrived? He's in Dr. Rabkin's office."

"I heard. I wonder what that's all about. What's he here for? Do you know?"

"I don't know the reason. But Mitch Rabkin brought him here, and there's a reason for whatever Mitch Rabkin does. Maybe it's to generate more attention to ethical issues. There are going to be some seminars."

"Well, if Dr. Rabkin is doing that, he must think the ethical issues are a growing priority. And maybe that's right. There are plenty of them in the background in my firm, anyway."

"I'd have to say the same. There's this case right now that's really tricky. Let me tell you about it. This guy comes into the ER, and he's obviously critical and wants treatment, but he refuses to be admitted. So we call psychiatry . . ."

I felt gratified that my presence alone, with the imprimatur of the hospital president, had catalytic effect independently of anything I had yet said or done. The message of that imprimatur was that ethical reflection is important; those two physicians had gotten the message and were already embarked on that reflection. This, too, was a part of learning medicine in Boston's Beth Israel. But sustaining and spreading that message remains a major challenge for medical education and practice.

10
· · ·
THE
LAST
VISIT

In October 1985, my wife and I went abroad for two weeks to celebrate our twenty-fifth anniversary. We returned from a joyful trip to find a chilling message awaiting us. J. Eric Nordlander, a close friend in Cleveland, was in serious medical trouble, as yet not clearly identified. In the weeks that followed, a dispiriting reality emerged. The diagnosis was of cancer, started in the intestinal tract, but metastasized to the liver and lymphatic system. The prognosis was bleak.

Eric was a productive organic chemist, a vigorous and distinguished educational leader, and a man of consummate candor and courage. He saw his plight for what it was, but resolved to take control of his situation and manage his care with the help of his physicians, rather than become a passive recipient of the decisions made by others. In this resolve, he was immensely supported by his wife Ruth, also a scientist of substantial accomplishment and, like many other family members of dying patients, a woman of grace and fortitude in the face of intractable adversity.

Humor had always been a part of Eric's life, and it remained an important part of his approach to his disease. He believed in its therapeutic power, and the capacity to laugh—and to amuse others—was with him nearly to his last breath. He adopted a severely restricted diet shortly after his diagnosis, in part on the basis of admittedly slim evidence about its possible benefits in retarding or arresting the disease process. But despite everyone's best efforts, his decline continued. Soon he had to leave his position as Dean of Arts and Sciences at Cleveland State University, a position he had occupied for less than eighteen months. Ruth continued to meet her faculty responsibilities at Case Western Reserve University, to care for the children, and to be companion, advisor, and nurse to Eric.

Shortly after the diagnosis, Eric had been hospitalized briefly. After that, he chose to remain at home. Hospitals, he concluded, were no place for the sick if there were any alternative. In this preference, as in the management of his case generally, he was sustained by the dedication of an extraordinary physician and friend from the Cleveland Clinic, Dr. Essie Esselstyn—a renowned surgeon whose last impulse is to do surgery. With Esselstyn's humane assistance, Eric stayed at home, surrounded by family and friends. By January, hope was fading fast. Eric and Ruth had read the relevant literature, studied alternate therapies ranging from guided imaging to drugs used abroad but not here, tried various combinations of approaches, diets, and medications, and witnessed the steady ravages of the disease.

The end came quickly. By February, it was clearly just weeks away. Jonathan Reichert, a physicist from the State University of New York at Buffalo and a close mutual friend, shared my frustration at the deteriorating situation. We resolved to create a program to honor the values that Eric held most dear. We wanted to involve him in its creation, both so that it would reflect his preferences in detail and so that its creation would enrich his life even as his death approached. I told Eric of this decision, setting him various related tasks.

As a loyal alumnus, he chose Cornell University as the site of the program, and selected the social responsibility of the scientist as its theme. Over the next few weeks, totally absorbed by the project, he spent much of his waning energy and many of his conscious hours designing that program to ensure significant undergraduate involvement with visitors of great prominence and social commitment. Within two weeks, enough contributions had been raised to endow the J. Eric Nordlander Visiting Scholar Program at Cornell.

Eric died at home on March 20, 1986, at the age of 52. At his memorial service, I said, in part:

I am here because Eric asked me to be. He raised the question of my speaking at this service in his characteristic way, making it easy for me, elevating me to his level. "You and I," he said, "are each at one time or another going to need a funeral service of some sort. And it's looking as if mine is likely to come first. I have some ideas about what I'd like it to be, and I wonder if you'd be willing to help out a bit." In the face of excruciating tragedy, there we were, two colleagues, talking together about one more subject of common concern. Only later did I fully realize how subtly and remarkably supportive of me Eric had been in what could have been such a difficult conversation.

He said he wanted nothing mawkish, but instead something more upbeat—a celebration of life. We told each other that day of what our friendship and association meant to one another. I emphasized that he was an uplifting model for me, not just in his presence, but in his absence as well. I told him of how, fighting one particularly unpleasant academic battle, I had thought of his unwavering integrity, and was sustained by the knowledge that he would have spurred me on had he been present. And I assured him that I would always benefit from this resource, whatever the outcome of his illness—that this was a part of his lasting legacy to me. . . .

Wondering how to honor that life, some of his friends noted his concern with the role of science in our future, his belief in the potential of leadership, and his dedication as a teacher. In establishing the program at Cornell that now bears his name, we sought to capture these central aspects of his agenda, so as to assure him that his agenda would be pursued in his name evermore.

We began in late February to raise funds to endow the program, and were able to confirm to Eric by mid-March that the program would be secure. The endowment still grows daily—a monumental tribute to how very much Eric has meant to a great many people, literally hundreds, across the land. Over these past three weeks, as news of the program spread, checks have cascaded in, large and small, from near and far. So too have letters and calls, testaments of love and admiration that filled Eric's final weeks

*with gratification and—I am convinced, despite his physical
decline—even moments of joy. . . .*

*He told me just two weeks ago that he found the whole project—
its prospects and the way its supporters rallied to the cause—so
redemptive as to make his medical problems seem comparatively
insignificant. . . .*

My close involvement with Eric Nordlander's dying at first
seemed unrelated to my encounter with Beth Israel Hospital. That
involvement was among the most intensely absorbing experiences I had ever had, overwhelmingly sad, yet richly rewarding.
From time to time, however, my thoughts returned to the patients
and families in the hospital. I thought again of Mrs. B, dying alone,
in terror and despair, of respiratory failure. I thought of old Mrs. T,
living on and on in the hospital, and wondered whether she could
remember an earlier life outside in the real world. I thought of the
elderly man sitting in the hall, shouting "Doctor Doctor Doctor
Doctor." I thought of the age-old question of what counts as a
good death, and realized that Eric, cut down at an early age by a
dreadful disease, had nonetheless achieved a good death as a
result of the nobility of his character and of how he brought it to
bear on his dying.

Central to the grace and power of that dying was a strong
element of control. Eric, with the assistance of others, was the
choreographer. He arranged to see his closest friends, often
delighting in the opportunity his illness provided him to introduce
to one another those he hoped would remain friends as a result. He
chose the music he listened to, the food he ate, the clothes he
wore. He even chose the music to be played at his memorial
service—jazz versions of traditional Protestant hymns. He completed letters of recommendation for his doctoral students. He
kept a schedule that suited him as well as possible in the circumstances—resting, visiting, telephoning, eating, thinking. He
could not forestall the relentless disease; short of that, to the end,
he was in charge.

How different it is in a hopsital! The physical surroundings at
best are starkly institutional. Patients are brought their meals at
mealtimes, not when they most feel like eating. Often, they are
given hospital gowns, designed for administrative convenience,

that denude them of their individuality and dignity. They typically have roommates, making genuine privacy impossible. Others, often strangers, come and go at will. The patient may be receiving an immense amount of genuinely caring attention, but has typically relinquished all but a few vestiges of control. If the patient is in intensive care, the level of control is diminished even further—and the patient in this context is not necessarily unaware of his or her plight. (In this regard, see Frederick Wiseman's extraordinary six-hour documentary film "Near Death," first broadcast on the Public Broadcasting System in January 1990, which provides a sustained and captivating view of treatment at the end of life in the Medical Intensive Care Unit of Boston's Beth Israel Hospital. It is, as the saying goes, the next best thing to being there.)

A dying patient has lost control over life itself, over the possibility of a future, over continuing to exist. This central fact can dwarf all others, making the psychological pain of dying more intense than the physical pain. If we care about the quality of life of those who are dying, we ought to be especially concerned to help them retain as much control as possible in every dimension of whatever remains of their lives.

The psychological importance of a sense of control over one's circumstances can hardly be overemphasized. Loss of control is among the most grievous burdens borne by prisoners, and wardens can manipulate prisoners with a structure of rewards and punishments comprising little more than modifications in the nature and number of choices over which the prisoners can exercise control.

From time to time, I have taught an undergraduate course on decision making. The goal is to study the difference between decisions that are made well and those that are not. The inquiry draws on work in cognitive psychology, operations research, philosophy, literature, and engineering. To capture the students' interest, I confront them with a question close to their hearts—how to choose which automobile to buy.

It is easy to persuade them that a formal method of analysis, such as one called a decision-matrix, offers the best hope of making a lastingly satisfying choice. That analysis structures their thinking, takes into account all the relevant factors such as performance, durability, price, comfort, and the like, and even gives appropriate weight to subjective considerations such as style and prestige. Soon, the entire class is sold on formal analysis.

At that point we turn to the high rate of failure in marriage. We read about arranged marriages in India, and consider the potential of computer-based expert systems to arrange marriages with a much higher success rate than unstructured individual choice. There is much skepticism about whether any computer-based system could actually play such a role, but that is not the point. The class is willing to imagine the possibility of a subtle, sophisticated, computer-based system that would work.

It might incorporate the results of an extensive interview, a probing psychological analysis, a personal history, and more. It would then match couples highly likely to have successful marriages, on the basis of principles derived from the prior analysis of tens of thousands of successful and unsuccessful relationships. It might work; assume for the moment that it does.

The important point is that even on the assumption that the system assures a very much higher success rate than any other method of mate selection, the students want no part of it. With few exceptions, even while granting that they are much more likely to have failed marriages as a result, they want to make their own choices. A successful outcome may be important to them, but control is even more important. They learn this fact about themselves with astonishment.

In a hospital, it is easy to become accustomed to the way the institution works. This is true of staff, visitors, and to some extent even of patients. It is easy to accept that things are done as they are because they must be done so for the hospital to function. In that context of acceptance, one can also easily overlook how pervasively patients lose control over important aspects of their lives, and how that loss of control crushes the human spirit.

One remedy, palliative at best, is to maximize the amount of control that patients retain in hospitals. There are limits to this approach because of the genuine needs of the institution, however. Another approach is to recognize the superiority of home care for many categories of patients, and to develop structures of financing and support that facilitate and encourage the return of the patient, even the uncomfortable patient, to the comforts of home.

Boston's Beth Israel, mindful of the importance of respecting the individual autonomy of patients, was first in the nation to adopt a patient's Bill of Rights in 1972. Its preface says, in part, "It is our policy to respect your individuality and your dignity. We support your right to participate in the decisions which affect your well-being." The ten basic points that then follow address such matters as the right to be addressed as one wishes to be addressed, to have one's questions answered, to be secure in the confidentiality of one's medical records and one's conversations with health care providers, and the like.

These are important protections, and do enhance the extent to which patients in the hospital maintain control. But it is still a hospital, and diminution of control is endemic to hospitals. That diminution is precisely what Eric Nordlander avoided, even as his body wasted away; that, perhaps, is why his intellect and his spirits could sparkle like jewels to the end.

Although there have been changes in health care since then, hospitals are still in the 1990s the same kinds of places—struggling to provide good care without financial collapse; striving to respect patient dignity despite the institutional constraints that prevent them from doing well; working to help all who come their way, knowing that the inadequacies of their knowledge and the mistakes that are an inherent part of their art will limit the good they can do. They are still good places to avoid when one can. And they can still be the best recourse one has.

It is Wednesday, February 22, 1988, at 4:45 A.M. Before the phone has finished its first ring, I am awake with the terrifying thought, "My father!" The call is from a house officer at the Beth Israel Hospital. She says that he was admitted some hours earlier, that he has had a respiratory arrest, that he seems to be having a major myocardial infarction, and that it would be a good idea for me to come to the hospital as soon as I can. The prognosis, she says, looks very bad. I ask for my mother; she gets on the phone. We talk briefly; I tell her I will be there as soon as the flight schedules will permit.

There is an early flight to Boston; I get a message to my mother that I will find her in the hospital by 10 A.M. At the airport I buy my ticket, look blankly at the clerk who has just wished me the automatic, utterly vacuous "Have a nice day," and head for the gate.

On the plane, I keep replaying a conversation with my parents the evening before, both on the line from Boston. My mother expressed concern that my father seemed to be coming down with a bad cold. His voice sounded thin and somewhat rasping; he had stayed home from his office, and was in some discomfort. "I got him to take an aspirin," my mother reported.

"An aspirin?" I replied. "Why not two?"

"One was all he would take," she answered.

"Now, you tell him," I admonished, "that if he is supposed to take two aspirin, then he had better take two, or I'll come up there to help you deal with him. I'll hold his nose so you can toss the second one in."

"You mind your own business," he quipped. "I can hold my own nose."

En route, I pictured the hospital, trying to visualize the Coronary Intensive Care Unit, hoping to get there faster by seeing it sooner. Questions flooded in on me: Is he still alive? Will he regain consciousness? Will I be able to talk to him ever again? How is my mother? How can I help? Will there be decisions that have to be made? What will I need to find out? Does my background help, or is it irrelevant now that I have to deal with a vital crisis, rather than just observe others doing it?

As my taxi approached the hospital, I realized how unusual it must be for someone rushing toward an ICU to feel as comfortably familiar with the surroundings as I did. I knew my way around this place. I knew the people and their values; I had heard them admitting their mistakes, affirming their aspirations, and bemoaning their frustrations. This, I realized, was where I wanted my father to be right now, and that seemed to me all at once the sum and substance of my view of Boston's Beth Israel.

By 9:15, I was in the hospital. I found my mother immediately, and her brother; I was found within minutes by various friends on the hospital staff. My father's condition was extremely bad. He was on life-support equipment, but his blood chemistry was terrible, his heart was working only with the aid of an external pacemaker, and his blood pressure, despite the use of drugs to elevate it, was distressingly low and falling. I learned to my relief that he had been conversant *en route* to the hospital, but had lost consciousness moments after arriving there, and hadn't regained it.

During that difficult day, my concern centered on the question of what possible level of functioning my father might sustain if he survived the acute crisis. He had always hated the idea of dependency and had steadfastly refused to consider retirement. I began not only to hope for a recovery but to fear one. By mid-afternoon it was clear that circulatory insufficiency had caused extensive damage, and that there was no possibility of a recovery of mental functioning. We agreed that DNR status was appropriate. At seven that night, he died.

I recalled a remark he had made a year or so earlier. "I'm not afraid of death. I just don't want to be around when it happens." In a sense, he wasn't. So he, too, had a death of the sort he seemed to favor. And he died "with his boots on," at eighty-two, having missed just a day or two of work, and having missed all of the dependency and deterioration that are so much a part of the dying of the elderly in so many cases. Hard on the family, to be sure, but not a bad ending, all things considered. I also recalled a discussion years earlier about what sort of death one would choose if it were a matter of choice; a colleague at a conference had responded, "On the golf course, at a *very* advanced age, immediately following a spectacular hole-in-one before a large group of admiring friends, by lightning from behind."

It was clearly a great advantage, on that last day at the Beth Israel Hospital, not only to have been familiar with the hospital, but to have thought hard and read and talked with many others about decisions at the end of life, about intensive care, about the treatment of the very ill elderly and the plight of the very dependent elderly, about how much is enough and how far is too far.

I had often argued that it is crucial for physicians to wrestle with difficult and challenging questions of value and judgment, and to confront their feelings about a variety of painful realities, on a hypothetical basis before having to confront them on an actual basis. Some medical educators have resisted that position, holding that until one must confront an actual decision or crisis, deliberation about such matters is mere speculation that has little impact—in part perhaps because one can never be sure how one will feel, and hence how one will act, before the fact.

Yet the impact of familiarity is profound. When the questions and realities that must be faced are recognized as the expected ones in such situations, they may still be as painful to address as if they were new and strange, but they can be less difficult. When one has thought and debated about the relevant issues, one has a reservoir of understandings, values, and positions to draw on in addressing the moment; one may find that the moment puts them to the test and possibly forces modifications in them, but one need not invent them on the spot in the context of crisis.

The point is completely general, of course. It has no special bearing on health care providers. Indeed, it is perhaps even more important for prospective patients and their families to be well informed and prepared to deal with mortal crisis than it is for young physicians. For physicians, unavoidably, will confront such matters again and again, and thereby will develop a perspective about them sooner or later.

For the rest of us, unless our lives are unusually beset by tragedy, such occasions will be few and far between. Yet, for that very reason, many of us tend to ignore such matters until they are upon us. Utterly absorbed in the pursuits of daily life, we can too easily avoid hard thought about such fundamental matters as the significance of family relationships, friendship, birth, illness, and mortality.

How lucky I was, as a philosopher, to choose a profession so thoroughly practical in regard to such centrally important aspects of life!

Following my return to Syracuse, I learned that condolences really do help. A great many kind people wrote, and many sought me out to talk. I was fascinated to see that they fell immediately into three sharply defined groups. The first group comprised those who expressed their sympathy—genuinely, but with no special stamp of personal involvement.

A second group contained those who had lost a parent themselves. One after another, they began by expressing their sympathy, and within minutes were talking about their own loss. That never seemed inappropriate; in fact, it was a welcome way of establishing a bond of common experience and common suffering. Yet I was struck by how rapid and universal the phenomenon was. It did not matter whether their loss had been just months earlier, as it was in some cases, or as long ago as in childhood, as it was in others. I was reminded of an oft-quoted remark about sightseeing in India: "The world is divided into two groups," the saying goes. "Them as has seen the Taj Mahal, and them as ain't." The world is also divided into those who have lost a parent, and those who haven't, and it took just minutes to tell them apart in a context of condolences.

The third group comprised people near to my age whose parents were living. Their sympathy for my loss was bound up with their own sense of vulnerability. In talking with someone from this group, I knew—again, in minutes—about their octogenarian parents—where those parents lived, what they did, whether they were well. I could see vividly how threatening one person's loss is to another who stands at risk of suffering a similar loss.

A nurse at Beth Israel Hospital has been a great help and comfort to my mother and to me during my father's final hours, which have ended just a short while ago. I speak with her briefly; then, she embraces me with tears in her eyes, and cries for a moment. "I'm sorry," she apologizes needlessly. "You see, my father is very sick."

Since leaving the hospital, I have had many occasions to think about my days there—about what I saw, heard, and felt, and about the lives of those who are patients or providers in the world of health care. One theme running steadily through those thoughts is the presence of uncertainty in health care—uncertainty about the physical realities, such as the proper diagnosis, the etiology of a condition, and the consequences of a contemplated intervention, and also uncertainty about the moral dimensions of the decisions that must be faced. It is these uncertainties that make it both necessary and so very difficult to draw the lines that are manifested in each decision about a complex and ethically challenging case. These uncertainties, and their endemic tenacity, also limit the utility of algorithms and make informed and sensitive judgment a continuing necessity in health care decisions. And the pervasive significance of these uncertainties, as much as anything, is essential to understand about contemporary health care if we are to deal well, as individuals and as a body politic, with the opportunities and problems it presents to us.

Each of us faces the need, over and over again, to decide how far to go in dealing with various dimensions of our lives. It may be a personal choice—about health care, allocation of resources, the use of one's time, or any of a great many other matters. It may be a question of public choice—about tax policy, aid to the disadvantaged, national security, or any of the rest. In either case, the decisions are most difficult when we lack both assurance about the factual aspects of the problem at hand, and also uncontested clarity about the values at issue.

Under such conditions, it is most useful to have reflected in advance about the questions and conflicts that must be resolved. Decisions that arise in and about any modern hospital often exemplify precisely this character. In trying to provide a sense of the experience of daily life in one such hospital, and in conveying the thoughts that were stimulated by my perceptions of that experience, I hope to facilitate reflection that can be brought usefully to bear on some of the difficult decisions that lie ahead.

ADDITIONAL
READINGS

The challenges raised by contemporary medicine and health care have captured the interest of the public, the various professions engaged in the provision and financing of health care, those involved at the levels of law and policy, the mass media, and the professional and academic literatures. The problem of recommending related readings is that they are readily at hand almost wherever one looks. This is a phenomenon of recent times, however. Twenty-five years ago, there was almost no discussion in the professional literature about ethical problems, nor were such discussions featured in the public media. Today they are ubiquitous.

As recently as 1975, the publishers of academic books were generally unwilling to consider works in medical ethics. The reasons were explicitly expressed; the publishers' inquiries confirmed that there was no such field, as evidenced by the almost complete absence of courses with any such subject matter. By 1980, courses in medical ethics had become part of the standard offerings at colleges and universities across the country.

Today, texts and anthologies related to the issues addressed in this book number in the hundreds. Many traditionally influential journals frequently discuss ethical and policy matters in health care. Among the most influential are *The New England Journal of Medicine, Annals of Internal Medicine,* and *The Journal of the American Medical Association.* In addition, many newer journals have a specific emphasis on these matters. They include, among others, *Medical Humanities Review, The Journal of Clinical Ethics, Ethics and Behavior, Bioethics Literature Review, The Journal of Medicine and Philosophy,* and *Hospital Ethics.*

The most central journal in this area, however, and the finest source of current information about the rapidly expanding literature, is the *Hastings Center Report* (available at libraries or from The Hastings Center, 255 Elm Road, Briarcliff Manor, New York 10510), now in its twentieth year. In each bi-monthly issue, a section entitled "In the Literature" provides annotated references to many of the most significant recently published books and government reports, plus articles from the relevant journals in law, philosophy, medicine, etc. The Kennedy Institute of Ethics (at Georgetown University, Washington, D.C. 20057), publishes the *Bibliography of Bioethics.* The recently published fifteenth (annual) volume contains more than 2000 citations, and covers court decisions and news articles as well as books and journals. This bibliography can be accessed through MEDLARS, the electronic information service of the National Library of Medicine.

Among the most significant government reports are the eleven reports published by the President's Commission for the Study of Ethical Problems in Medicine and Biomedical and Behavioral Research (Washington, D.C.: U.S. Government Printing Office, 1981–83). At the state level, among the leading reports are those of the New York State Task Force on Life and the Law (Third Floor, 5 Penn Plaza, NY, NY 10001), covering a wide range of topics. Several volumes providing a variety of international perspectives are published by the Council for International Organizations of Medical Sciences; these are available through the World Health Organization (Avenue Appia, 1211 Geneva 27, Switzerland) or through their book sales agents. Quarterly reviews of writings and issues in medical ethics in Great Britain, often with iconoclastic commentary, appear in the *Bulletin of Medical Ethics* (6 Galia Road, London, N5, England).

INDEX